THE
Natural Guide
TO
Colon Health

THE
Natural Guide
TO
COLON HEALTH

LOUISE TENNEY, M.H.
with Deanne Tenney

WOODLAND PUBLISHING

Pleasant Grove, UT

© 1997
Woodland Publishing, Inc.
P.O. Box 160
Pleasant Grove, UT
84062

TABLE OF CONTENTS

INTRODUCTION

Digestion is the power source of body energy. The fuel is the food we eat. Energy comes from nutrients found in the food—vitamins, minerals, enzymes, amino acids, carbohydrates and lipids. These nutrients allow the body to perform many vital functions that literally keep it alive. All nutrients and sources of energy are vital, though different amounts of each are necessary. If the wrong foods are eaten or toxins are ingested, the body will not be able to work properly.

Digestion involves the important and essential functions of assimilation and elimination of food. If assimilation is not proficient, valuable nutrients will be lost. If elimination is insufficient, toxins can be reabsorbed into the bloodstream, which can lead to many disorders. Thus we see that when the digestive process is working well, the body is generally in a healthy state.

In our less-than-ideal world, there are daily opportunities to come into contact with toxic substances. The air we breathe, the water we drink, and the food we eat all contain some level of toxic material. This makes it even more important to concentrate on a healthy diet with supplements to aid the body in removing waste. If the body is in optimum shape, it is better able to deal with the bombardment of toxins.

In the past, medical doctors focused on the health of the colon as a requisite of overall health. But, unfortunately, with passage of time and with advancements in medicine, some of the most basic medical concepts are now overlooked. One of these forgotten fundamentals is that disease is related to colon health. The idea behind this entire book is that a healthy colon is the basis of a healthy body. Learning natural methods to achieve colon health can be of great importance. Nutritious eating habits, cleansing diets, herbal remedies, and nutritional supplements can all contribute to total body well-being. A healthy body requires a healthy colon.

OVERVIEW OF CHAPTERS

Chapter One
PAST PERSPECTIVES ON DISEASE AND THE COLON

Looking to the past will only help us in the future. Many medical professionals in the past looked to the colon first and were able to treat various health conditions with excellent results. In this chapter we discuss some early research and results, and present a great deal of information about basic colon health. Several important physicians and their contributions to the field are introduced with the hope we can learn from their experience.

Chapter Two
CONSTIPATION: A NEW DEFINITION

Constipation means many things to many people. Some individuals may even be constipated and not know it. This chapter will help you identify problems of constipation, why they occur, and how to overcome them.

Chapter Three
DISORDERS ASSOCIATED WITH THE COLON

Many syndromes and conditions are related to colon health. Allergies, candida, hernias and leaky gut syndrome are possible results of colon problems. If we are aware of the reasons behind our illnesses, they are much easier to cure. It is important to always remember to treat the colon when dealing with disorders. Once the colon is healthy, other symptoms will disappear.

Chapter Four
THE IMPORTANCE OF FIBER

A lack of fiber in the diet is an important factor in constipation and other colon disorders. Many conditions seemingly unrelated to colon health have been linked to a lack of fiber in the diet. We explain how fiber affects the body and look at specific types of fiber. Included are recipes that will allow you to introduce fiber into your diet in a tasty, enjoyable way. We finish the chapter looking at many specific disorders and diseases that are related to lack of fiber.

Chapter Five
NUTRITIONAL KEYS TO IDEAL HEALTH

It is necessary to understand the key nutritional needs of the body and how deficiencies can affect health. Most people are not aware of the importance of an acid/alkaline balance in the body, so we discuss that subject at length. The importance of fats, enzymes, amino acids and acidophilus are also discussed as prerequisites to overall general health.

Chapter Six
CLEANSING PROGRAMS FOR A HEALTHY BODY

Cleansing the body helps to keep every system working properly. Body systems work together and need to be kept clean and healthy to function efficiently. This chapter provides specific suggestions about how to cleanse the various body systems and organs, including the use of herbs and supplements.

CHAPTER ONE

PAST PERSPECTIVES ON DISEASE AND THE COLON

While no one will dispute the marvels of medical technology and its amazing ability to transplant organs, repair massive injury and perform incredible surgical feats, the fact remains that modern medical practitioners may have actually regressed in their assessment of what really causes disease and how to best heal the body. In other words, in our rush to abandon obsolete, outdated medical practices for the latest pharmaceutical drug or sophisticated diagnostic machinery, we may have inadvertently overlooked the basic and necessary keys to health and well-being.

I. HISTORICAL VIEWS OF COLON HEALTH

DR. ARBUTHNOT LANE

In 1929, Dr. Arbuthnot Lane, a well-respected English physician and colon specialist, made the dramatic statement that constipation was the cause of all ills of civilization (Jensen 1982, 408). Dr. Lane had worked for years as a surgeon; naturally he continually dealt with bowel problems. His hands-on experience with repeatedly removing sections of diseased intestinal tracts provided him with impressive data, along with a first-hand look at the profound role of the colon in overall health. One of the most striking correlations he discovered was the link between a malfunctioning colon and seemingly unrelated diseases. He noticed this particular phenomenon when some of his patients, who were recovering from colonic surgery, experienced remarkable cures in other parts of their bodies that had no apparent connection to the colon.

A young male patient of Dr. Lane's had suffered from such serious arthritis for several years that at the time of his colon surgery he was confined to a wheelchair. Six months after the colon surgery, he experienced a complete recovery from his arthritis. Another female patient who suffered from a goiter showed signs of remission within six months of her colonic surgery. Dr. Lane was intrigued by these results and subsequently discovered a long list of diseases, ranging from tuberculosis to rheumatism, which were cured when certain diseased sections of the person's bowel were removed. More specifically, he found that there was a correlation between specific areas of the colon and certain body organs.

Dr. Lane was so impressed with the notion that a toxic bowel can determine the health of other body systems that he completely changed his methods of medical treatment. Through his study of scientific evidence, he discovered that the relationship between the bowel and the maintenance of a healthy body was an intrinsic one. Because of his conviction that proper care of the colon was essential for the prevention of disease, he spent the last twenty-five years of his life dedicated to teaching people how to care for their colon and how to avoid the risk of bowel surgery through proper nutrition. He emphasized the importance of transit time (how long waste material is retained in the colon) when he said, "The lower end of the intestine is the size that requires emptying every six hours, but by habit, we retain its content twenty-four hours. The result is ulcers, cancer and other diseases" (Jensen 1982, 408).

Dr. Lane believed in the supreme value of nutrition. He taught that "all maladies are due to the lack of certain food principles, such as mineral salts or vitamins, or to the absence of the normal flora. When this occurs, toxic bacteria invade the lower alimentary canal, the poisons generated pollute the bloodstream and gradually deteriorate and destroy every tissue, gland and organ of the body" (Jensen 1982, 408).

Dr. Lane was not the only physician of his time to emphasize maintaining a healthy colon. Investigating the medical literature of the early part of the twentieth century discloses that many medical doctors recognized the colon as a significant cause of disease. Unfortunately, their provocative research and writings are hidden in old, dusty archives and rarely come to the attention of the current medical establishment. Following is a brief overview of some of their findings.

DR. JOHN KELLOGG

When attempting to evaluate or treat disease, most physicians rarely explore an individual's colon health. An exception was Dr. John Harvey Kellogg, a colon specialist who maintained that 90 percent of the diseases of civilization are due to an improperly functioning colon. For forty years, Dr. Kellogg studied the health of chronic invalids by X-raying their colons and observing their surgical procedures first-hand. He discovered that in hundreds of these patients constipation had developed because of poor diet and a lack of colon hygiene. He also found that in the majority of cases, chronic constipation was curable without resorting to surgery. Kellog felt that through diet alone the colon could be stimulated to function in a regular and efficient manner without the use of harsh laxatives or drugs.

DR. BERNARD JENSEN

Dr. Bernard Jensen is modern-day physician who has done extensive research into the findings of many earlier doctors. He explains that after treating over 350,000 patients of his own, he discovered "every organ and tissue is dependent upon the health and well-being of every other organ and tissue in order for there to be total well-being" (1982, 12). In other words, no organ is an island. He goes on to say, "If there is a faulty functioning in the bowel, this deficiency is passed along to the rest of the body. We literally poison ourselves into illness in this manner" (1982, 407-8). While it may sound rather ominous, the role of the colon cannot be overestimated.

DR. HENRY A. COTTON

While researching articles published in the *Journal of the American Medical Association,* we located several pieces of literature discussing the use of colon cleansing and its successful outcome. In particular, a 1932 article reviews the research of Dr. Henry A. Cotton, a physician who performed autopsies on the colons of insane patients for several years and discovered one or more problems affecting the bowel. The article states:

> . . . an examination of each specimen reveals one or more of the following characteristic changes in the bowel: 1) destruction of the epithelium and mucosa; the mucous membrane may be denuded and eroded over large areas, there may be edematous thickening of the muscular wall and congestion of the peritoneal coat; 2) areas of hemorrhage, pigmentation and ulceration; 3) extreme atony and atrophy of the muscular coats with the bowel wall thinned places to a parchment-like consistency, resulting in dilated, pouchy areas referred to by Cotton as "segmental blowouts;" 4) marked thickening of the bowel wall due to chronic fibrous tissue growth; 5) adenitis (inflammation) of the mesenteric glands (this was invariably present); and 6) the presence of diverticulosis. In addition, Cotton discovered that in every instance, cultures taken after surgery or as postmortem procedure from the enlarged mesentery lymph nodes found in colon and small intestine tissue, contained various types of streptococci and virulent colon bacilli." (Synnot, 441)

What Dr. Cotton had observed was a phenomenon called autointoxication (discussed in Chapter Two). Simply stated, autointoxication refers to the poisoning of body systems through toxins, carcinogens and other putrefactive waste material which is harbored in the bowel and subsequently allowed to reenter the circulatory system through the intestinal walls. The following section deals with the notion of bowel toxins and how they affect health. It more than aptly illustrates the fact that physicians of the early and mid-twentieth century were well aware of the dangers of bowel poisons.

Colon Toxicity

In 1909, Dr. J. A. Stucky, M.D., presented some valuable findings at a meeting of ear, nose and throat physicians. He explained how the colon is related to the danger of autointoxication:

> The question of intestinal autointoxication, toxemia and lithemia has at last come to the front where it belongs, and has gained wide attention from the medical profession, both in Europe and America, and the results and treatment of putrefaction and toxemia originating in the intestinal canal have become matters of great importance not only to the practician, but to the otorhinologist. Unsatisfactory results obtained after months of surgical and local treatment of some diseases of the ear, nose and throat have stimulated a more careful search for reasons why permanent relief was so rarely obtained from usual accepted and time-honored methods of treatment. In several hundreds of cases of diseases of the nasal accessory sinuses, middle and internal ear in which surgical interference and operative procedure were resorted to, I have found unmistakable and marked evidence of toxemia of intestinal origin as evidenced by excessive quantity of indican in the urine, and when the condition causing this was removed, there was marked amelioration of entire relief of the disease . . . Toxins, owing to disturbed body chemistry are manufactured daily in the intestinal canal and remain in the system; the result is a pretest from irritated nerves and poisoned cells, manifested in rheumatic pains, asthmatic attacks, vertigo, obscure necrosis of eye, ear, nose and throat, neuralgias and periodic headaches; all these being evidence of systemic poisoning. This poison I have almost invariably found to be the indican in the urine. (1184-85)

It is important to remember that physicians of the early twentieth century were aware of the profound role a malfunctioning colon played in disrupting homeostasis, or good health. In 1929, Dr. Robert B. Osgood, M.D., read a paper before the American Orthopedic Association in which he described a patient who happened to be another physician with Type 1 rheumatoid polyarthritis, also known as toxic or infectious polyarthritis. After eradicating all possible sources of infection from the teeth, tonsils, sinuses, genitourinary tract, etc., Dr. Osgood related the following:

> We attacked a sluggish intestinal canal by methods of severe purgation by drugs and enemas as advocated by Jones of New York, whose writings and successes were then attracting attention. We employed, in addition, the correction of his body mechanics and what we believed to be a rational dietary and fresh-air regimen for over a month without avail. His disease progressed. We finally told him that we believed his disease was so far advanced that we were helpless. He made arrangements to return to his home permanently crippled. A few days before he was to leave the hospital, without additional therapy except, I believe, abdominal massage and more through colonic irrigation, he suffered a huge, quite unexpected movement of his bowels, consisting of dark, very offensive, obviously very ancient material and began at once to have less pain in his joints. The articular and periarticular swelling subsided with surprising rapidity and after a few months of out-of-doors life and a few manipulations to break up adhesions, he resumed his practice and has continued in it ever since. When his joints give him warning, he resorts to irrigations of his colon and he reports himself as well, happy and quite satisfied with life.

Dr. Anthony Bassler, M.D., was well acquainted with the phenomena of reabsorption and colon congestion—two physiological events that most of our modern-day physicians know little about. In 1941 he said:

> Many of the most toxic individuals that I have seen have daily and often more frequent bowel movements. Only by the sensation of satiety that comes from complete colon emptying or

by X-ray methods can normal function for the individual be judged. One must keep in mind that hyper-transit through the intestine may come from irritation and congestion and that mild degrees of this may exist in the constipated individual in this way moving the bowels more normally. In constipation, the use of purgative remedies usually increases the toxemia by way of induced congestion and increased reabsorption (21-22).

These accounts are dramatic, to say the least, and much of their value lies in the fact that they came from credible, intelligent medical practitioners. These doctors supported the notion that all systems of the human body are intrinsically interconnected. With their observations, research and study, these doctors prove that the condition of the colon can be a predictor of health or disease.

High-Protein Diet

Regarding our obsession with high-protein diet and colon health, medical practitioners knew decades ago what is only beginning to reemerge today. Eating an excess of protein can cause autointoxication. While it may seem perfectly normal for feces to have an unpleasant odor, the fact remains that bowel movements with an unusually offensive smell are not inevitable. In other words, what you eat can determine to a great degree the level of putrefaction of your waste. In 1930, Dr. William E. Fitch published an article titled *Putrefactive Intestinal Toxemia*. He states:

> The putrid decomposition of proteins is universally repugnant and substances undergoing this change are, beyond question, decidedly unfit. All putrid matter is toxic. It would appear that Nature in her wisdom willed that putrescence carries with it a foul odor, warning both man and animal that such material is unfit. Experience emphasizes the fact that putrid food is poi-

sonous and is capable of producing, and does produce, poisonous toxins which are absorbed into circulation. Moreover, clinical observation emphasizes the fact that putrefactive decomposition in the intestinal tract is capable of, and where present, does liberate poisons and toxins that are absorbed into the circulation with the most deleterious and harmful results. (183)

Dr. Fitch goes on to describe a whole host of symptoms produced by intestinal toxemia, including headache, lassitude, mental and physical hebetude, anorexia, coated tongue, fatigue, weakness, insomnia, neurasthenic weakness and even melancholia.

The Colon and Eye Disorders

Today we rarely hear of physicians linking colon toxicity to eye disorders. Unquestionably, the idea that eye disease may be initiated by intestinal poisons would seem rather radical to modern-day medical practitioners. Yet in 1914 the notion was apparently perfectly reasonable. That year Dr. Clark W. Hawley, M.D., delivered a paper before the Chicago Ophthalmological Society. In part he stated:

The making of the diagnosis of lower bowel fermentation of an abnormal character is not difficult, but the two facts which stand out most prominently are 1) that it is hard to cure and takes much time and patience on the part of the doctor and the patient, but when properly done, the reward to both are ample, and 2) that the lower bowel should be the source of toxins which leave their evil manifestations in the eye is not so very remarkable when we consider that it is here that the waste food products are stored, and if not promptly discharged, their toxins are being absorbed into the circulation. Nature provided a large organ to destroy them, but its capability is limited and the surplus continues on in the circulation; at some point

21

it finds a tissue properly prepared to receive it, and there it starts its deadly work. In the eye, the uveal tract is, on account of its exceeding vascularity, a very good stopping point for any wandering toxic material. So we have iritis, cyclitis, irico-cyclitis, choroiditis, and other inflammatory manifestations. (663-74)

While the language may sound rather old-fashioned, the content is based on sound science. It is worth noting that in his discussion of the colon and the eyes, Dr. Hawley may have also inadvertently explained why working with the bowel was eventually abandoned by modern-day doctors. In his own words, it "takes much time and patience on the part of the doctor and the patient," two commodities our society has little of.

Dr. Hawley goes on to relate his own personal experience with eye disorders and eating protein. Once again, he supports the notion that the decomposition of protein in the bowel creates poisons which can affect seeming far removed organ tissue. He explains:

. . .while still on a strict diet, I was taking my meals at the club and eating pie for dessert, this all of the month of February, 1913. On the first of March, I began to be bothered with the opacities (vision obstructions) again and tried hard to think in what manner I was overstepping my instructions and found it was a good-sized piece of cheese with each piece of pie. I cut out the cheese and in a month it disappeared. My eyes remained free and my urine would show only a mere trace of extractives. On the first of January, 1914, I decided to try a very moderate protein diet in the way of meat, as on a strictly vegetable diet one does not have the energy he does on a mixed diet and ate sparingly during January and February. In March, I noticed the same old opacities obscuring my vision again. I at once commenced treatment, confining myself to a strictly vegetable diet, and at this time, April 20th, 1914, the opacities are hardly perceptible. This and the cheese incident show you that one must not eat the least of protein food while the bowel is throwing a large quantity of extractives into the circulation. One must keep to the vegetable diet until a new and healthy condition is established before going back to a mixed diet, and then he must commence cautiously, feeling his way along. Absolute abstinence must be the law. (19)

By now, it should be obvious that many medical practitioners of our century openly acknowledged the role of toxic colons in determining health. The physiologic method by which bowel poisons are reabsorbed into the body is addressed again in an article by Dr. Martin J. Synnott, published in the *Medical Journal and Record: A National Review of Medicine and Surgery*. Consider the following quote:

> As a result of the invasion of the colon by pathogenic bacteria, virulent toxins are produced. The mucosa of the bowel is irritated by the toxins or invaded by the microorganisms themselves. Absorption takes place through the lymphatics and capillaries of the colon. The bacterial poisons eventually act on the nerve supply of the abdominal organs causing spastic colitis, or contributing to the production of atony and atrophy of the muscular coats of the bowel, with delayed motility, constipation and stasis. (441-446)

Here the role of pathogenic bacteria in the colon is discussed. Most of us are aware of the vital importance of maintaining a healthy intestinal bacterial flora. Unfortunately, if the diet is poor and the colon sluggish, harmful bacteria flourish and contribute to more putrefaction and toxicity. To make matters worse, we rarely replenish our intestinal flora by eating good sources of acidophilus (live bacteria), and we routinely kill our own friendly bacteria by the excessive use of antibiotics, other drugs, a poor diet, alcohol, etc. We inadvertently create the perfect environment for pathogenic bacteria to flourish and thereby make our bowel more toxic than ever.

Clearly, physicians of the past were well aware of the phenomenon of autointoxication. What about today? Are these concerns addressed in the doctor's office or at hospitals? Sadly, much knowledge concerning colon health has fallen by the wayside, abandoned for the "quick fixes" of pain killers, antidepressants, antibiotic drugs and scads of over-the-counter laxatives. What we can learn from Dr. Arbuthnot and his contemporaries is that if you are sick, look to your colon first. Most physicians would probably be unaware that you may be suffering the aftermath of autointoxication. Unfortunately, very few physicians will be asking you about your bowel habits, so you need to do some learning and investigating on your own. This book will help. Learn how the colon works, and learn about changing your diet, using herbs and cleanses, and getting enough exercise. Determine for yourself if the condition of your colon has health-determining power. If you do these things, we guarantee that you will become a believer in the importance of a healthy and a clean colon.

II. NATURAL LAWS OF HEALING

The law associated with healing is known as "Herring's Law," in honor of Constantine Herring (1800-1880), a 19th-century European homeopath physician who is considered the father of American homeopathy. Herring's Law states, "All cure comes from within out, from the head down and in reverse order as the symptoms have appeared in the body." To understand this, we can break the law into three parts.

First, Herring states that when when the body is involved in the natural healing process, symptoms tend to move from the deeper parts of the body toward the surface. Flu-like symptoms may develop; skin rashes and eruptions may appear on the mucous membranes of the nose, mouth, and vagina; a runny nose, diarrhea, or an infection may appear. These are signals that the body is trying to eliminate the disease outward. The symptoms may come from emotional, mental, or physical problems, but whatever the cause, these symptoms are part of the healing process. They need to be allowed to occur naturally without suppression by drugs or heavy foods.

Second, when the body is being healed naturally or is undergoing a cleansing program, symptoms tend to move down the body from the head to the feet. An example is a rash that will move from the face to the chest to the abdomen to the thighs. Other symptoms like muscle cramps or joint pains may move from the shoulders to the hips and then to the legs and feet as healing occurs.

Third, previous symptoms that were suppressed in the past, or incompletely cured, may return—usually in the reverse order of their original occurrence. The symptoms could be from childhood or they could be from a suppressed condition from ten or twenty years ago. Even a sore throat that was experienced as a child, if suppressed, could appear in the healing process. The last symptom that occurred will probably reappear first, whether it be bronchitis, flu, headache, sinusitis or any other condition. Disease can be stopped by antibiotics and other medications that suppress the symptoms, but the toxins remain in the body and become solidified.

Another part of the process is that, as natural healing takes place, the symptoms tend to move from more vital to less vital organs or body symptoms. For example, as depression begins to clear, a heart flutter may develop. Then it will clear up but there may be heartburn or digestion problems.

Disease often takes many years to manifest, and renewed health has to be earned by improved diet and lifestyle. A whole new way of thinking and living needs to be learned. This "reversal process" is nature's way of righting what was wrong in the body. It is nature's way of protecting, healing and strengthening the body.

Chronic disease, acute disease and cleansing fasts can all benefit from the use of natural products such as herbs. They help clean the body through natural processes and aid the body in cleansing itself. The cleansing herbs help to neutralize toxins in the body. Red clover blends are excellent sources to aid the cleansing process. Colon herbs help to rid the body of toxins through the digestive system. Strengthening the nervous system with nervine herbs can help open the channels of elimination, cleanse the blood and build up the vitality of the body.

Benefits of an Improved Diet

One of the greatest misunderstandings in the field of nutrition is the failure to properly understand the symptoms and changes that take place when beginning a better nutritional program. What happens when foods are introduced in the diet that are of higher quality? When adding more grains, beans, fruits, vegetables, nuts, seeds, sprouts and juices, what happens in the body? When we begin to concentrate on foods that are in their natural, unrefined forms, what changes can we expect? What occurs in the body when we eliminate chocolate, coffee, tea, alcohol, tobacco, sugar and white flour products from the diet?

The higher the quality of food added to the diet, the quicker the body recovers from disease. Using the proper food combinations can help with cleansing and healing. The most easily digested foods should be eaten first, the more complex second, and the most concentrated last. Higher quality food allows the body to discard old tissue and rebuild healthier tissue.

Headaches are one of the most common symptoms that occur when an individual is eliminating foods such as coffee, tea, soft drinks, cakes, cookies, chocolate and all sweet junk food from the diet. The headaches occur because the body is trying to discard toxins that have been removed from its tissues and transported through the bloodstream. Before the toxins are eliminated, they will irritate different areas of the body and cause symptoms like headaches and depression. They may even stimulate a cold, but this is just nature's way of cleaning the body.

Stimulants (like caffeine) and other toxins can cause a rapid heartbeat and produce feelings of exhilaration. When these toxins are eliminated, the body experiences a let-down and the slower action may cause a depressed state of mind. This usually occurs within three days of the elimination and may last a few days, but once the symptoms vanish, the body will be stronger and have more energy than it did before.

Do not abandon an improved diet until you give it a real chance. If you go off it too soon, you may not want to return because you felt better on the old diet. It is important to give the body a chance to go through the cleansing process and adjust to the changes. After about the first ten days, the vital energies which are usually in the muscles and skin begin to move to the vital internal organs and reconstruction begins. This will reduce energy in the muscles and may cause feelings of weakness so it is a time when the body needs to rest. In fact, a change in diet or a fast should only be undertaken when you have time to rest and relax. Your body is using its energy to detoxify on a cellular level.

As higher quality food is eaten, the body begins to go through a process called *retracing*. This is when the body is ready to "clean"—to get rid of toxins and excess bile from the liver and gallbladder and eliminate those toxins through the intestines. The arteries, veins and capillaries begin to move sludge and eliminate it from the body. Deposits in the joints begin to clear out. The tissues begin to eliminate waste, and they discard it more rapidly than new tissue can be made. This is the phase of cleaning when weight loss may be noticed.

Stabilization occurs when weight loss basically stops. The amount of waste being discarded daily is equal to the amount of new tissue being formed. Anabolism happens next. Weight begins to increase even with a lower calorie diet. This happens because new tissue is being formed at a faster pace due to improved assimilation made possible by the discontinuance of poor eating habits and the wrong combination of foods. Increased energy can be expected at this point in the process.

Be aware that symptoms which have been suppressed in the past may appear when following a nutritional program. Colds that have not run their full course may arise. If an individual has a tendency for skin rashes, these rashes may emerge. This is the body's way of eliminating toxins through the skin. The skin is throwing off the long-deposited poisons and becoming more active and alive. The result is ridding the body of these poisons before they can cause more serious disease. Such elimination may save the body from liver damage, kidney disease, blood disease, arthritis, nerve degeneration or even cancer. The symptoms are merely a part of the healing process.

III. ACUTE DISEASES

While disease is usually a strong warning that health habits need to be changed, some acute diseases are actually a friend to humankind. Various acute conditions such as colds, influenza or inflammation allow accumulated poisons to be eliminated from the body. Many times disease provides the primary means of toxin elimination from the body and is a natural cleansing process. Nature provides the body with this built-in cleansing mechanism, but it is sometimes misinterpreted as negative because it manifests itself in the form of acute disease.

Dr. Henry Lindlahr, a medical doctor in the early 1900s, was considered an expert on this subject. His fundamental laws of cure, which form the basic principles of the science of natural healing, clearly illustrate that acute disease is itself a cure. Dr. Lindlahr taught that an acute disease represents the body's efforts to purify and regenerate the system.

What is an Acute Disease?

Acute diseases have a rapid onset and run a short course. The period of distress and discomfort of an acute condition is quite brief as compared to a chronic disease which lasts for a long period of time. All acute diseases are based on nature's law of curing—that is, the body tries to rid itself of toxins and promote a cure. Scientists around the world have spent billions of dollars seeking a cure for the common cold. They want to find a drug that destroys the virus that causes colds. Hopefully, this will never happen. We need to understand that all acute diseases, including the common cold and the flu, are a cure for whatever toxic condition the body is trying to overcome. These acute diseases are nature's effort to eliminate waste, toxins and poisons from the body and to repair damaged tissue. Every acute disease is a cleansing process and healing effort. Acute diseases include all childhood diseases such as asthma, bladder infections, croup, diarrhea, dysentery, ear infections, eye infections, tonsillitis, colds and influenza.

In summary, acute diseases have a rapid onset and usually run a short course. They are a natural cleansing which eliminates germs, toxins and foreign material from the body. Suppressing the symptoms may lead to chronic conditions at a later time.

COMMON ACUTE DISEASES

- appendicitis
- bladder infections
- Bright's disease
- chicken pox
- congestion of the kidneys
- croup
- diarrhea
- dysentery
- endocarditis (acute)
- eye infections
- German measles
- gout (acute)
- hay fever
- hives
- influenza
- laryngitis
- mumps
- phlebitis
- pneumonia
- syphilis
- tetanus (lock jaw)
- toothache
- tuberculosis
- asthma (acute)
- boils
- bronchitis
- colds
- coughs
- cystitis
- diptheria
- ear infections
- enteritis (acute)
- gastritis
- glaucoma
- gonorrhea
- hemorrhages
- hydrophobia
- jaundice
- lung problems
- nephritis (acute)
- pleurisy
- scarlet fever
- smallpox
- tonsillitis
- typhoid fever
- whooping cough

TREATING ACUTE DISEASES

Again, colds, flu and fevers are part of a natural eliminative process. They are a safety valve which the body opens of its own accord to give itself a chance to eradicate toxins. A short fast will help hasten the stage of acute disease. When experiencing an acute disease, use lemon, lime, grapefruit and orange juices diluted with pure water, as well as herbal teas. No sweet juices such as grape or apple should be used during an acute disease as they cause fermentation in the intestinal tract.

Essentially, an acute disease is a healing and cleansing of the body as it attempts to eliminate accumulated toxins and poisons from the cells and organs. It brings them to the stomach to be eliminated, but the cleansing process is stopped when food is eaten. The stomach has to use its energy to digest instead of cleanse, so the body is depleted of the healing energy. The irony is that people usually feel better when this natural cleanse is stopped because their aches and pains go away for a while. This reprieve in symptoms is deceiving, however, because all that is really happening is that the mucus and toxins are being driven deeper into the body. It will take an even greater cleanse to get rid of them the next time.

Dr. Lindlahr and Natural Laws

Why do people catch colds after they are chilled? Dr. Henry Lindlahr explains why in his book *Philosophy of Natural Therapeutics.*

Taking cold may be caused by chilling the surface of the body or part of the body. In the chilled portions of the skin the pores close; the blood recedes into the interior, and as a result, the elimination of poisonous gases and exudates is locally suppressed. This "catching cold" through being exposed to a cold draft, through wet clothing, etc., is not necessarily followed by more serious consequences. If the system is not much encumbered with morbid matter and if the kidneys and intestine are in fairly good working order, these organs will assist the temporarily inactive skin to take care of the extra amount of waste and morbid material and eliminate them without difficulty. The greater the vitality and the more normal the composition of the blood, the more effectively the system as a whole will react in such an emergency and throw off the morbid material which were not eliminated through the skin. (174-5)

Dr. Lindlahr taught some wonderful concepts about natural laws. He proved in his medical practice that all acute diseases are the same in nature and purpose and that they run the same course through five stages of inflammation. These stages are: incubation, aggravation, destruction, abatement and reconstruction. All five stages are necessary for complete cleansing and subsequent healing of the body. Every disease, whether it is acute or chronic, has to go through these five stages of inflammation. This is a law of nature.

Some people think that they are healthy because they never get sick, yet they have improper diets and allow stress to bind them up. These people need to initiate a cleanse by going on the same program as those who come down with acute diseases. Persons who eat devitalized foods and go year after year without a cleansing may someday develop a full-blown chronic disease and wonder what possibly could have caused it.

Five Stages of Disease

INCUBATION STAGE

The first stage of disease is the *incubation* stage. This describes the period when the inner body is accumulating toxins, poisons, drugs, toxic metals, pesticides and inviting germs to accumulate. The toxins accumulate in the tissues, causing an obstruction at any of various places in the body. This is also the period when vitality and energy in the body will be low, and the body will be under stress. The energy and nutrients of the body are depleted due to stress, personal problems, poor eating habits and the pressures of life. The body is unable to fight off the invading germs, viruses and bacteria. This period may last for several days, weeks, months or even years.

AGGRAVATION STAGE

The second stage is the *aggravation* stage. This is the stage when the battle between the immune system and toxins is waging. When toxins have accumulated to such an extent that they interfere with the normal functions of life or endanger the health of the body, the life forces begin to react to the obstruction. This results in inflammation and, as the condition progresses, it may be accompanied by fever and congestion. This is when symptoms appear and we begin to realize that we are getting sick. If medication is taken to relieve the symptoms or the toxins are not eliminated, the cleansing process will be stopped and the toxins and mucus will bury themselves further into the organs of the body. They can build up in the joints, the lymphatic system or anywhere else in the body. They can accumulate around organs such as the heart and veins and may solidify, leading to a chronic condition.

DESTRUCTION STAGE

The time when the body is trying to fight against invading germs, viruses or toxins is referred to as the *destruction* stage. This stage may be accompanied by a corresponding increase in fever and inflammation, and is usually when the crisis peaks. Excess waste is eliminated along with built-up chemicals, fatigue and harmful emotional acids. The body is cleansing itself of toxins before they become hard and difficult to remove. This is the stage when it is necessary to let nature cleanse at its own pace (it may even end in crisis, depending on the energy level and vitality of the individual).

When the destruction stage of an acute disease is suppressed, the organs remain permanently damaged. This is the stage when a large amount of pus and mucus is created in the body due to the old tissues being broken down. The organs will be holding the mucus and toxins. If the elimination process is halted by medication, the pus, mucus and other toxins may remain in the organs and could lead to more serious conditions such as pneumonia, tuberculosis, spinal meningitis, asthma, emphysema or bronchitis.

ABATEMENT OR ABSORPTION STAGE

The fourth stage, referred to as the *abatement* or *absorption* stage, involves excess waste being eliminated from the body. The battle against disease is being won by the body. The right form of treatment builds the blood and immune system, increases vitality and promotes natural elimination. Glands in the body, primarily the lymphatic and intestinal glands, absorb the excess waste. As that occurs, the fever will abate and other symptoms will decrease. As natural healing processes continue, the toxins will be expelled from the body. But if this cleaning up stage is suppressed, the toxins will be thrown back into the body. The glands are filled with toxins so suppression can develop into conditions such as lymphatic congestion, glandular secretions, tumors, cysts, moles and skin disease.

RECONSTRUCTION STAGE

The fifth stage is the reconstruction stage. When all the other stages have run their course, rebuilding may begin. The affected areas will have been cleared of the toxic accumulations and obstructions. Cells, tissues, blood vessels and organs that may have been damaged will begin to regenerate.

If the reconstruction phase is interfered with or stopped before it is complete, the toxins will continue to invite germs and other toxins to the affected areas of the body and the organs will not have a chance to become entirely strong and clean. The body will remain in a weakened and diseased state, unable to function properly. This will lower the immune system and the glands will remain full. They will swell and shrink and will be unable to produce hormones properly. As a result, there may be a low hormonal output, low lymphatic absorption and the intestinal tract may still be coated causing indigestion, anemia and nutritional deficiencies. This will cause a build up of toxins and lead to chronic diseases that may be incurable such as cancer, candida, diabetes, herpes, Epstein Barr virus and many more.

Negative Emotions

Some individuals eat a very nutritious diet and follow what they assume to be a natural approach to health, but still suffer from some forms of toxic conditions in the body. It is important to remember that negative emotions breed inside the body and will affect the function of the body. Stress can upset the organs, glands and turn food eaten into toxic substances. Hate is such a strong emotion that it can wreak havoc with the body and cause turmoil inside, producing toxic acids. Negative emotions will jeopardize the immune system.

Stress can cause even more damage if the body is in a compromised position due to a diet high in junk food and poor eating habits. A positive attitude will help improve the health of the body. No one can avoid the stress that comes with life, but we can build the immune system to combat the negative emotions. Proper bowel management, cleansing, nutritional foods, and a positive mental attitude will contribute to a longer, healthier life.

IV. DISEASE CRISIS OR HEALING CRISIS?

The Healing Crisis

While carrying out a colon cleanse you may develop what is commonly referred to as a healing crisis. A healing crisis is telling you that your body is trying to eliminate toxins, and by doing so may cause distress of one kind or another. A healing crisis appears as the body is going through a process of elimination by ridding the body of toxins and drugs. The disease crisis is when the body is full of disease and cannot function well but is still attempting to eliminate and heal the body. The healing crisis is a natural cleanse that occurs because of the individual has implemented some form of a cleansing diet. The body needs to be in good enough shape to hold up during the process.

It may take a few months after changing the diet for the healing crisis to occur. It usually lasts only a few days, with symptoms including headache, fever, cold, flu, or diarrhea. Some individuals may eliminate the toxins more gradually and will not suffer the severe symptoms. It is important to remember that the body is undergoing a process of elimination. Feeling bad for a few days is very common in the healing crisis. Don't give up the effort.

TIPS FOR DEALING WITH A HEALING CRISIS

• Rest if you are tired. The body needs extra energy to heal.
• Drink liquids when thirsty and eat only when you are hungry.
• Fruits are cleansers and eliminate toxins and can sustain the body with their natural sugar, vitamins and minerals. If you are cleansing too "fast" on fruits, slow it down by including steamed vegetables, vegetable juices or vegetable broths.
• Vegetables are higher in carbohydrates and will slow down the cleansing process. This may be needed when the body needs to be strengthened and built-up in order to go through another cleanse.
• Herbal teas can be used.
• Avoid mucus-forming foods.
• Avoid alcohol, caffeine, tobacco, coffee, tea, chocolate, white flour products and sugar.
• Herbs, vitamin C complex and other supplements help the body to dissolve mucus and toxins. Blood cleansers, colon cleansers, chlorophyll, or blue-green algae are some agents that will help remove obstruction and congestion in the body. Enemas may be needed when the colon is congested.
• Massage therapy will speed the cleansing process. Foot reflexology will help eliminate and break up toxins.
• Chiropractic treatments will help the body heal faster.

SYMPTOMS OF A HEALING CRISIS

• Food cravings
• Diarrhea
• Sore throat
• Insomnia
• Sore muscles/leg cramps
• Depression
• Fever
• Headaches
• Skin rashes
• Nausea

- Change in menstrual cycle
- Discharge from nose, eyes, bowels or urinary tract

Healing the body will bring positive results such as a feeling of well-being, less cravings for junk food, reduced desire to overeat, better circulation, clear skin, more energy, freedom from pain, improved digestion and the elimination of disease.

SUMMARY OF A HEALING CRISIS

1. A healing crisis may happen when the body is naturally cleansed through fasting or semi-fasting using wholesome and nourishing food.
2. A healing only happens when the body has enough vitality to withstand the cleansing symptoms.
3. A healing crisis usually occurs when the body feels its best.
4. A healing crisis usually develops about three months after a change in diet or fasting.
5. The healing crisis can last from two to seven days. If the vitality of the body is low, it could last longer than a week.
6. No crisis may appear if correct eating, along with colon and blood cleansing eliminate the waste a little at a time.
7. The body goes through three stages in order to completely clean the body—eliminative, transitional and building. The crisis will usually manifest during the transitional stage.
8. A chronic disease may cause aches and pains as the body is discarding toxins. The chronic disease took years to develop, and may take a small cleansing crisis to overcome. The pain during a healing crisis may be more severe than when the the chronic disease was developing.

Some people may want to give up when they start experiencing the worst part of the healing crisis. They do not understand what is happening to their bodies. If they take drugs, the disease is stopped, but it is pushed deeper into the system to manifest itself later in symptoms of a more advanced disease.

The Disease Crisis

A disease crisis happens when the body becomes congested with built-up toxins. Germs, viruses, parasites and worms can invade and the body ceases to function properly. This is when nature takes over and forces the body to eliminate. In cases of colds, flu and fever, the body is attempting to cleanse and restore health naturally to a toxic body. These are acute diseases and should be treated naturally with fasting, juices, and herbs. Acute disease should not be suppressed with drugs and heavy foods, which stop the cleanse and may push it deeper into the body. An acute disease needs to run its course naturally.

A disease is produced not only when the body is overloaded with toxins and mucus, but when constipation develops and when the strength vitality of the body is lowest. Remember that negative thoughts and emotions increase toxins and prolong their stay in the body. Emotional stress can very well cause a disease crisis. And as difficult as it may be to accept, a disease crisis happens in order to protect life. If the congestion continued at the rate it was increasing, it would cause damage to the vital organs and could develop into chronic diseases such as cancer, heart disease, or asthma.

STRESS AND DISEASE

Stress can cause disease by dilating the capillaries. Dilation causes the pores in the capillary walls to enlarge. The vessel walls can become hard, brittle and give out. The enlarged pores allow the blood proteins to pass from the capillaries into the tissues between the cells. This causes an imbalance in minerals and symptoms of disease increase. Stress causes the organs to tighten up and prevents the natural process of digestion, assimilation and elimination.

When all is said and done, we all know that a healthy body is important for a quality life. The quality of our life can also influence the health of our body. It is hard to really enjoy life if we are always ill or under extreme stress. By changing some old habits for new, our quality of life can be greatly improved. Just remember that any changes should be made gradually.

CHAPTER TWO

CONSTIPATION: A NEW DEFINITION

The simple fact that a tremendous number of people suffer from constipation conveys a profoundly clear and succinct message—whatever it is that we are choosing to eat or not to eat is affecting our colons in a negative manner. There is no question that the human machinery we call our body is a marvelously designed bio-unit designed to function efficiently. Ideally, it ingests food, chemically breaks down the components of the food, absorbs nutrients for energy and cellular regeneration, and finally expedites waste to the large intestine where it should be expelled in a relatively short amount of time.

This step-by-step system is the optimal way the body was meant to operate. The mere fact that chronic constipation disrupts this sequence of ingestion and elimination is a signal to us that something is seriously wrong. While the miseries of constipation are well known, its health implications are not.

Not eliminating waste properly can negatively affect virtually every other body system. Moreover, constipation involves much more than just failing to have a daily bowel movement. Many of us are unaware of the fact that we are probably suffering from some form of constipation. The health implications of impaired elimination are profound, to say the least.

Medical practitioners rarely emphasize the very vital role that proper elimination plays in determining how we feel, the probability that we will become sick, our mental health or even the likelihood of premature death. The general consensus is that constipation is just constipation and simply requires the use of a laxative. Basically, most of us think, it's no big deal. Unfortunately, this widespread view could not be more inaccurate. Constipation, especially chronic constipation, is a big deal and should be treated with sound nutrition and natural therapies rather than with harsh chemicals.

Before we go on, it is vital to determine whether we are actually suffering from constipation. Surprisingly, many of us who consider ourselves to be "regular" may discover that in reality, we have been constipated for long periods of time. Contrary to popular belief, just having a regular bowel movement doesn't mean that everything is as it should be.

Here is a perplexing question: How often should a person have a bowel movement to be considered healthy? This query will usually spawn a variety of answers ranging from after every meal to four times per week. The current technical definition of constipation refers to a decrease in bowel movements or difficulty in the formation or passage of the stool. While this definition may be technically correct it is incomplete and fails to explain all of the ramifications of a dysfunctional colon.

In reality, several kinds of constipation exist and most of us unknowingly suffer from one form of this malady or another. John Harvey Kellogg, M.D., in his book *Colon Hygiene,* describes three forms of constipation:

Simple Constipation: This condition is seen when the elimination of the bowel content is not complete. Consequently, fecal matter remains in the bowels and gradually builds up and adheres to the colon wall. This condition can result from irregular eating, overeating cooked food, lack of exercise and neglecting the urge to eliminate. This may signal the beginning of chronic constipation and may be involved in the cause of over 90 percent of the diseases plaguing mankind.

Cumulative Constipation: This is considered the most common form of constipation. It is mostly confined to the lower part of the colon and is due to lazy peristaltic action. The purpose of peristaltic waves is to propel the contents of the colon from the cecum to the rectum for eventual elimination. Lack of normal bowel action can cause injury to the colon walls and the ileocecal valve. Consequently, straining is usually necessary to eliminate the bowels. This straining can eventually cause hemorrhoids (internal and external), varicose veins, lower back pain and many other symptoms.

Latent constipation: This type of constipation typically occurs in people who suffer from chronic disease. Latent constipation takes years to develop and most people are not aware of its presence because the bowels move regularly (1978, 195-200). Symptoms of this kind of constipation are numerous and include: fatigue, headaches, bad breath, appendicitis, colitis, PMS, anxiety, and depression. The list could go on and on.

I have added a fourth form of constipation which may seem like a contradiction in terms—diarrhea. Diarrhea can often be a type of constipation. Dr. John Christopher says that "diarrhea is simply a bad condition in the intestinal tract, where it is so badly clogged that the fecal solids are being held back and only the eliminative liquids are getting through." In other words, diarrhea is caused by an irritation or obstruction in the colon. Chronic diarrhea can occur when certain irritants adhere to the bowel walls and cannot be eliminated. In these cases, an herbal lower bowel formula will help to peel off any hardened bowel residue.

Naturally, not all cases of diarrhea signal constipation. Diarrhea may be caused by food poisoning, parasites, intestinal flu, colds, anxiety and a number of diseases such as ulcerative colitis, Crohn's disease, diverticular disease, irritable bowel syndrome or cancer of the large intestine. When an infant experiences diarrhea, it is vital to treat it promptly to prevent dehydration. Replacing lost electrolytes must be immediately addressed. Older people can also become dehydrated if chronic diarrhea is a problem. In any event, it is important to realize that some forms of unexplained diarrhea may be the result of incomplete elimination and may respond to treatments designed for constipation.

I. CONSTIPATION—THE CAUSES AND SYMPTOMS

Constipation can be caused by a number of factors and should really be considered more of a symptom than an actual disease. American bowel patterns are not statistically impressive and this supports the notion that our diets are deplorably low in fiber. It is important to acquaint ourselves with all the possible causes of constipation because its presence can lead to all kinds of miseries and ailments.

We must keep in mind that what goes in does not always come out. Recently, the notion that you can have regular bowel movements and still be suffering from constipation is receiving more attention. This idea is based on the fact that even when we have a regular bowel movement, it may not be a complete one. What this implies is that waste residue can build up on the walls of the colon and is never properly excreted when bowel muscles contract. In other words it "sticks," thereby leading to the development of bowel disorders and various other diseases.

While an earlier section discusses various reasons why we may develop constipation, the greatest cause, by far, is a dietary one. It is a well-established fact that typical American eating habits promote constipation. Americans purchase more laxatives that any other nation on earth—in the United States alone, annual sales of laxatives and stool softeners amount to over $500 million annually. That fact has profound health implications for our society. You can be certain that the topic of regular bowel movements is rarely discussed in cultures where dietary fiber intake is high. In many of these societies, constipation has never existed. But in the United States it is a source of major concern.

Great segments of our population have become severely addicted to laxatives. Western diet and lifestyle have resulted in the acceptance of constipation as a normal liability of living. The vast amount of over-the-counter laxatives consumed by our population not only cause dependence but may actually perpetrate the problem, not to mention its vitamin-depleting side effects. Unfortunately, many of us will continue to put up with the miseries of constipation when it can be cured by simply changing our eating habits and employing some very effective natural remedies.

Lack of fiber, combined with eating large amounts of mucus-forming foods, causes the body to produce excess amounts of mucus in order to protect the gastrointestinal tract from damage or toxin absorption. An abnormal build-up of this digestive mucus can slow transit time, thus causing bowel contents to remain in the colon much longer than they should. As a result, more moisture is absorbed from waste matter and eventually it becomes hard-packed, often adhering to the bowel wall. When an excess of fat and white flour products are consumed, a glue-like substance is created which readily sticks to the walls of the colon. In time, this gooey residue will harden and build up layer after layer, becoming a stiff, rubbery material. Pockets in the colon will collect this hard material and prevent its elimination from the bowel.

Causes of Constipation

• A lack of dietary fiber
• Bowel adhesions due to infected or deranged mucus membranes of the bowel wall
• Stretched colon from food overload
• Ileocecal valve incontinence, which allows bowel content to reenter small intestine and subsequently causes body system damage
• Lack of exercise
• Drinking too little water. Dehydration can cause fecal matter to become hard and prevent its complete elimination.
• Poor posture can interfere with the voluntary and reflex contractions of muscles
• Hemorrhoids can cause spasms or tightness of the anal muscle, which can prevent normal bowel evacuation
• Weak bowel muscles can prevent the complete emptying of the colon, allowing fecal matter toxins to irritate mucus membranes and produce chronic catarrh (mucus), infections, adhesions and even cancer
• Nervous disorders can cause tension in the bowel, thereby tightening the colon and anus
• A lack of hydrochloric acid and digestive enzymes can lead to constipation and autointoxication

In addition to the above causes, constipation can be caused by pregnancy, neurological and endocrine disorders, diabetes, an underactive thyroid gland and medications. Some of these drugs include codeine, antacids with aluminum, iron tablets, and some narcotics and antidepressants. Stress and anxiety have also been linked to constipation. A physical obstruction in the bowel caused by a stricture, tumor or diverticulosis may also result in constipation. An enlarged prostate gland or the presence of endometriosis may put pressure on the rectum, subsequently decreasing bowel activity.

II. AUTOINTOXICATION: A VERY REAL THREAT

Autointoxication is a term which refers to becoming poisoned from our own body contents. It occurs when the bowel does not function properly, and has been referred to as the root of numerous diseases which currently devastate our society. Poor eating habits coupled with lifestyle stressors, pollution, etc., cause the bowel to experience faulty elimination. This creates an encrusted colon, full of unexpelled fecal material. As mentioned earlier, this waste matter provides the ideal breeding ground for all kinds of undesirable bacterial strains and puts an enormous strain on the immune system. When the immune system is overly taxed, resistance is compromised and opportunistic infections move in. A constant battle with colds, flu, sore throats, yeast infections etc. may be a signal that the colon is perpetrating infection.

In addition, a heavy mucus coating which can form in the colon (and which will be discussed in the next section) becomes putrid and full of poisonous compounds. The tiny blood capillaries that nourish colon tissue can pick up these poisons and transfer them into the bloodstream; hence, the term "autointoxication." Several different kinds of carcinogenic and deranged hormonal compounds may be among these toxins and may influence the development of various cancers, hormonally induced diseases, autoimmune diseases, and even the process of aging itself. Some of these chemicals include:

- bile salts
- heavy metals
- pigments
- poisons

- volatile fatty acids
- deranged hormones
- preservatives

Eating a diet that is high is protein is a special cause for alarm. Protein is more difficult and takes longer to digest. If the colon is impaired protein can turn into a number of very deleterious chemicals. Undigested protein and its by-products may be much more detrimental to the human body than previously thought and may help to explain why so many diseases are on the rise in Western cultures.

In short, constipation may be a much more serious condition than our physicians would have us believe. To say that it may play an intrinsic role in the health of virtually every physiological body system is not an overstatement.

III. SYMPTOMS OF CONSTIPATION

- painful bowel movements due to the hardness of the stool.
- inability to have a complete bowel movement.
- bloating and gas
- tender or distended abdomen
- feeling of sluggishness

- development of hemorrhoids
- indigestion
- insomnia
- depression or anxiety

Excess Mucus in the Body

Interestingly, when cooked foods are eaten, large amounts of mucus are secreted. Foods that are particularly mucus forming include meat, cheese, milk products, pastries, candy, white flour products, white pasta and all processed, refined foods. These foods may appropriately be referred to as "glue foods." Nature provides mucus as a protective coating which surrounds gluey material to keep the intestinal membranes from absorbing toxic substances.

We are learning that when cooked food is eaten, the T-cells, which are so vital to immune function, increase in the gastrointestinal tissue to protect our system from certain foods which are interpreted as foreign matter. If we consume cooked and processed food day after day without adequately eating raw food and fibery foods, protective mucus will form in excess and build up on bowel tissue similar of the age rings we see in the trunks of trees. Dr. Bernard Jensen, in his book *Tissue Cleansing Through Bowel Management*, writes,

> Mucosal dysfunction occurs when the intestinal mucus lining becomes stagnant and putrefactive. It begins to develop many unfavorable conditions. No longer does it serve the function of facilitating elimination of fecal material. Instead it degenerates in several ways. It can become abscessed, in which case irritations, abrasions, ulcerations and bleeding can occur. Food passage can be very painful. Mucus can dehydrate and accumulate due to increased viscid consistency. This causes layer upon layer to be built up until extreme constipation occurs. This old

material becomes a source of infection and toxic absorption, holding many otherwise excreted products. It also greatly inhibits the absorption of nutrients and water, adding to nutritional crisis. (39)

As a result of faulty eating, nature's protective coating—which was designed for occasional use only—becomes deranged and inadvertently contributes to ill health. Consequently, the immune system is taxed and the presence of this excess mucus creates a perfect medium for the multiplication of bacteria, viruses, parasites and worms. Autoimmune diseases may develop due to the fact that the immune system has begun to attack the body, rather than invading microorganisms. Continually eating "lifeless" foods—cooked, refined or processed foods devoid of fiber and enzymes—overstimulates the immune system in a way that compromises its function. As a result, we become susceptible to every virus and bacteria, constantly coming down with sore throats, colds, flu or other more serious conditions we may not think to relate to our digestive systems.

IV. PREVENTING CONSTIPATION

After reading the previous material on why constipation can be so detrimental to overall health, one may ask the question: what exactly can be done to prevent constipation? Adding fiber to your diet in combination by eating plenty of raw fruits and vegetables can work wonders. The amount of fiber recommended for anyone who suffers from constipation is 40 grams per day. Cereal sources of fiber combined with certain fruits and vegetables is highly recommended. Remember to increase your water intake anytime your fiber consumption goes up. The following are recommendations designed to prevent constipation:

- Before eating breakfast, drink a glass of fresh lemon juice squeezed in warm water
- Avoid all junk foods, white flour, rich dairy products, fried foods, sugar, coffee, alcohol
- Emphasize whole grain foods, peas, apples, cooked dried beans, oatmeal, raw nuts, soaked figs, prunes, plums, raisins, dates, fresh rhubarb, and okra
- Chew food completely, and don't overeat
- Eating directly before going to bed is discouraged
- Drink plenty of pure water, and keep a pitcher of water with lemon or lime in the fridge at all times
- Exercise regularly
- Take an acidophilus supplement regularly
- Use appropriate herbs when necessary

In summary, constipation is a very serious health threat with far-reaching consequences. It is a common but very dangerous malady that afflicts every segment of our society. Bowel dysfunction can manifest itself in many ways; however, the bottom line (no pun intended) is that a clean and efficiently functioning colon is absolutely essential to our health, well-being and longevity.

CHAPTER THREE

DISORDERS ASSOCIATED WITH THE COLON

I. ALLERGIES

An allergy is a condition that occurs when the body overreacts to a foreign substance. The immune system is actually responsible for the allergy because it misinterprets common, usually harmless elements as threats. It mistakenly attacks invaders such as dust, pollen or food. This causes an an allergic response which triggers antibodies to produce histamines, amine compounds which cause inflammation and lead to watery eyes, itching, sneezing, or other symptoms. An allergic reaction can result from something eaten, inhaled, or touched, and allergic sensitivities can occur at anytime during an individual's life.

It is often hard to pinpoint the exact allergen (the thing causing the allergy), but symptoms such as inflammation, pain, swelling or redness will probably accompany exposure.

Be aware of your environment and food and don't overlook the obvious. Allergic reactions can appear anywhere in the body—it's not always sneezing or puffy eyes. Reactions can also vary greatly in their severity. Some people suffer only minor irritation during hay fever season while others are allergic to the point of going into shock. Hives, asthma, digestive disorders, fatigue, nosebleeds, and food intolerances are just a few of the symptoms associated with allergies.

Irritation such as skin contact with chemicals, itching eyes from pollution and coughing due to exposure to cigarette smoke are not considered true allergies. Carolee Bateson-Koch, a well-known expert on allergies, gives some information on recognizing an allergy.

> The greatest challenge with allergy is recognizing it. We have been conditioned to think of allergy as being limited to such symptoms as runny eyes, sniffling nose, sinus problems, skin rashes, asthma and hay fever. However, allergy is much more insidious and extensive. It can also take the form of arthritis, gall bladder disease, intractable headache, Chron's disease, depression, psychotic behavior and more than one hundred other conditions not normally thought of as allergy. Allergy does not cause every disease, but it can be involved in almost any disease. It can play an integral role in the development of disease. It is so prevalent that if you have not been told the cause of your health problems or symptoms, you should consider allergy first. (7)

Allergies are not usually considered as life-threatening—after all, who ever died from a runny nose? The truth is, however, that allergies can be very serious. A condition called anaphylaxis, a massive allergic reaction that kills in minutes, is altogether too common. Few other diseases can kill so rapidly. Anaphyaxis kills within sixteen minutes to two hours after contact with an allergen, whether it be from a bee sting, a handful of peanuts or a penicillin shot. It is important to recognize and deal with an allergy in order to help improve your health and the quality of life.

Causes of Allergies

Allergies are a disorder of the immune system. They occur due to an imbalanced and weakened immune system response to poor diet, polluted air, chemicals or other toxic substances. There is usually not just one cause but a variety of factors that precipitate the condition. This can make allergies difficult for doctors to diagnose, and they often end up treating only one symptom with drug therapy which often masks the true problem.

The colon plays an important role in the prevention of allergies. Irritations from environmental pollutants, foods and certain plants can cause a weakening of the mucous membranes in the body, making them more permeable and allowing toxins to enter the bloodstream. (This is what happens to people suffering from leaky gut syndrome.) Food and toxins that make contact with the lining of the digestive tract can cause irritations and sensitivities.

Other colonic problems are associated with eating a lot of junk food, sugar, meat, and nutritionally poor food. These, along with all the toxins in the environment, can cause the colon to become congested or constipated. If this occurs, toxins can reenter the bloodstream and lower the immune system, setting the stage for allergies.

Toxic overload combined with frequent exposure can cause a weakening of the immune system and lead to the development of allergies. Most individuals are exposed daily to toxins such as pesticides, automobile fumes, chemicals and industrial pollutants. Over a period of time this can cause serious problems with the immune system. If the system is weakened, allergies can result whenever the body encounters certain foods, environmental pollutants, pollens, pets, dust mites or insect venoms.

Why some individuals are more susceptible to allergies than others is difficult to determine. The tendency to become allergic to foreign substances can be passed from parent to child, so there is a genetic predisposition in some cases. It has also been found that babies who have been breast fed suffer from fewer allergies. Formula-fed babies are more likely to develop allergies. It appears that mother's milk contains some protective antibodies. Stress may also be a factor in developing allergies. Stress, anxiety and prolonged emotional problems can lead to a compromised immune system.

Many of the common diseases in the United States are associated with a poor diet. Nutritional inadequacies contribute to various forms of illness. In her book *Allergies,* Carolee Bateson-Koch states,

> Eating a diet high in fat, sugar and refined, processed foods alters normal digestion. Digestion is the cornerstone of nutrition. It is also a cornerstone to understanding allergy. When you eat food, it goes through a series of chemical breakdowns called digestion. Proteins break down into amino acids, carbohydrates break down into glucose and fats break down into fatty acids. When this breaking down fails to happen, symptoms occur. When foods are fully digested, they enter the bloodstream in the normal way. The body recognizes them as nutrients and utilizes them accordingly. If they are not in the correct form when they enter the bloodstream, the body recognizes them as foreign invaders and attacks as if they were viruses or bacteria. (82)

It is clear that diet plays a vital role in allergies. The digestive system needs to be given the tools to work properly. If the system is not functioning due to a number of factors, the whole process can be in danger. Avoiding foods that create an allergic reaction will help to relieve symptoms but will not effectively deal with the underlying problem. Eliminate possible foods for four weeks. Reintroduce those foods one at a time. Do not eat foods that contain little nutritional value.

Symptoms of Allergies

- hives
- inflammation
- itching
- sneezing
- sinusitis
- constipation
- arthritis
- depression
- nervousness
- lethargy
- excessive gas
- colitis
- belching
- indigestion

- rashes
- watery eyes
- nasal congestion
- runny nose
- diarrhea
- irritable bowel syndrome
- headache
- withdrawal
- irritability
- hyperactivity
- nausea
- canker sores
- heartburn
- eczema

Dietary Guidelines

- A cleansing diet can help to eliminate toxins from the blood.
- Digestive enzymes and hydrochloric acid can help with the digestion and absorption of food.
- Juice fasting with carrot, celery and raw apple juice may be beneficial.
- Colon cleansing using gentle herbs can help with constipation.

- Make sure the liver is healthy by using a liver cleanse. The liver is responsible for ridding the body of accumulated toxins. It also helps to produce histaminase which protects the body against allergies.
- Avoid foods with additives. Stay away from FD&C yellow #5 dyes, along with BHT-BHA, benzoates, annatto, eucayptol, monosodium glutamate and vanillin.
- Eliminate foods that cause allergies; these often include wheat, eggs, dairy products, caffeine, chocolate, shellfish, strawberries, tomatoes and citrus fruits. After approximately four weeks, the foods can be reintroduced one at a time. Stay away from foods that offer no nutritional value.

Nutritional Supplements

Acidophilus: Acidophilus helps maintain a healthy intestinal flora. It also helps to eliminate undigested proteins.

Calcium with Magnesium: These help to reduce immune stress often created by allergens. They protect the body from allergens and reduce the inflammatory response.

Coenzyme Q-10 and Germanium: These help to stimulate immune response and improve oxygenation.

Digestive Enzyme Combination: Enzymes are necessary for digestion and every chemical reaction in the body. Digestive enzyme deficiencies may contribute to allergies.

Multi-Mineral Vitamin Supplement: A good multi-mineral and vitamin supplement will help strengthen and protect the immune system.

Potassium: Potassium is helpful for adrenal gland function and for muscle and nerve impulse.

Quercetin: This is a bioflavonoid that helps to increase the immune response.

Tyrosine: Tyrosine is an amino acid used to treat allergies caused by grass pollens.

Vitamin A and Beta Carotene: These help to heal and strengthen the mucous membranes. They also work as antioxidants to protect the body from free radical damage.

B-complex Vitamins: The B vitamins are important for digestion and nerve function. They help the body deal with stress.

Vitamin C with Bioflavonoids: This combination works as an antioxidant to protect the immune system. It also helps to maintain cell and tissue health, which can be compromised due to histamine release.

Herbal Supplements

Bee Pollen: Bee Pollen helps strengthen the immune system and build up a gradual immunity to some allergens. Start with a small amount and increase gradually. Discontinue use if a rash, wheezing or other symptoms develop.

Blessed Thistle: This helps to loosen mucus and strengthen lung tissue.

Burdock: Burdock works as a blood purifier to clear toxins through the lymphatic system.

Echinacea: Echinacea is another natural antibiotic and immune builder.

Ephedra: This is good for nasal and chest congestion.

Garlic: Garlic is a natural antibiotic and helps by fighting infection.

Goldenseal: Goldenseal fights infection, improves digestion and aids in the absorption of nutrients.

Kelp: Kelp provides essential nutrients and strengthens the body.

Lobelia: Lobelia acts as an expectorant to move mucus or obstructions in the body. It helps to relieve spasms that may occur in the bronchiole tubes.

Marshmallow: Marshmallow helps in relaxing the bronchial tubes.

Pleurisy Root: Pleurisy root helps to thin and loosen mucus and facilitates the elimination of toxins through the pores.

II. AUTOINTOXICATION AND THE NERVOUS SYSTEM

The health of the colon is essential for a healthy body. Many medical doctors in the past, as well as some health-oriented doctors today, know that the health of the colon can determine the health of the mind and the nervous system. Autointoxication, namely in the forms of toxemia and constipation, can lead to nervous disorders.

How does the nervous system fit into the development of disease? The symptomatology of the nervous system in connection with chronic intestinal toxemia is divided into four classes, namely cases involving (1) the mental system, (2) the sensory system, (3) the motor system, and (4) the sympathetic system. We have yet to find a case in which there was not present some involvement of the sympathetic system, but in some cases this is much more pronounced than in others.

The symptoms that are most characteristic and directly attributable to irritation of the sympathetic system are: (1) the cardiac symptoms, including rachycardia and palpitation; (2) peripheral vasomotor symptoms, such as diminished blood supply to the skin and resulting dry, brittle hair and nails; (3) gastrointestinal symptoms, including disturbances of taste and smell, appetite, nausea, vomiting, changes in secretion of the digestive juices, constipation and diarrhea; and (4) disturbances in the endocrine system, with hypothyroidism, hyperthyroidism, and alteration in the secretion of the suprarenal and other glands of internal secretion. The nervous system is almost invariably affected by chronic intestinal toxemia and the nervous symptoms are often the most prominent of the symptomatology.

Dr. Bernard Jensen, D.C., N.D., made the following statement in his book *Iridology, The Science And Practice in the Healing Arts*:

> In my experience, it is evident that what comes into the nervous system by way of the senses and by way of our emotional responses is just as important as the biochemical balance of nutrients we take into the body. Just as there are healthy foods and junk foods, there are healthy experiences and junk experiences. The nervous system is the center for consciousness, memory, intelligence, thinking, reasoning and emotions. The system is constantly monitoring the internal and external environment and adjusting the body functions to maintain a state of equilibrium. (298-99)

The sympathetic nervous system is rightly named for it is in perfect sympathy with the emotions. Tension, anxiety, worry and stress all cause problems with digestion and assimilation. This in turn can lead to malnutrition and accumulation of toxins; ultimately, disease can occur.

The sympathetic nervous system can become over-stimulated by emotional strain caused by tension, worry, fear, hate, anxiety or depression, among other things. The sympathetic and parasympathetic systems govern the functions of the digestive system. Any emotional trauma will disrupt and throw the sympathetic nervous control out of balance. If the body is in good health, it will bring the body back into balance with little problem. But if the body is laden with toxins, there will be further strain and disruption of the nervous system.

The sympathetic nervous system has a contracting and astringent action. The parasympathetic system has an expanding and relaxing action. The sympathetic side of the balance results in a strong contraction and tightening of the membranes and glands, such as the stomach, small and large colon, and adrenal glands. If the internal tension continues, it can lead to a chronic condition. The glandular secretions are changed by continuous internal stress affecting the secretion of enzymes. This tension also interferes with the small and large intestine's ability to absorb nutrients.

When the body is under extreme stress, the body can become malnourished even though an individual is eating well. The contents of the small intestine pass undigested material into the colon, which has only limited ability to absorb nutrients. If the irritation continues on the stomach and small intestine, a leaky gut syndrome can develop and cause allergies along with autoimmune diseases. When this material reaches the large colon, it is not able to receive undigested material and begins to reject it. This puts the colon out of balance, causing it to tighten up. Nutrients, moisture and minerals are not properly absorbed.

Emotions can directly affect the health of the body. Thoughts and feelings need to be positive in order for the body to work at its best. Positive thoughts stimulate blood flow and increase dilation of the arteries and capillaries. The digestive system will not work properly if the sympathetic nervous system is not in balance. Sorting out and coming to terms with emotional upset will help the body stay healthy and fit.

With emotional distress the stomach becomes irritated and different conditions may develop such as ulcers, colitis, or appendicitis, and the glands may become weakened and malnourished. When the stomach tightens up, the blood supply is unable to reach every cell of the membranes, and less blood will reach the stomach lining. This can cause congestion and inflammation of the stomach as the blood does not nourish the stomach lining. If this is allowed to continue, the cells will die from lack of nourishment. When the cells die, putrefaction occurs and the dead white blood cells form pus, then ulcers and eventually may lead to cancer.

A common condition that sometimes results from nervous disorders but is also the cause of many nervous disorders is constipation. Constipation may be an underlying cause of some cases of depression, mood swings, despair, stress, anxiety, insomnia or even strokes. In his article *Chronic Intestinal Toxemia,* published at the turn of the century, Dr. Anthony Bassler shows that physicians have long realized such effects. "Many of the most toxic individuals I have seen have daily and often more frequent bowel movements. In constipation their use of purgative remedies usually increases the toxemia by the way of induced congestion and increased resorption" (160).

In June 1917 the consequences of constipation were further discussed at an annual session of the American Medical Association. Three physicians, in their article *Symptomatology of the Nervous System in Chronic Intestinal Toxemia,* reported that 518 cases of mental symptoms ranging from mental sluggishness to hallucinations were relieved through eliminating intestinal toxemia (Satterlee, 1414). Research such as this leaves no doubt as to the serious conditions that can result from constipation.

Noteworthy research looking at the correlation between constipation and strokes is currently underway in China. In fact, statistics in China have shown constipation to be one of the most common symptoms in ischemic stroke. Chinese healers often treat stroke by looking for and treating constipation. As for the cause of stroke, along with constipation

Chinese physicians include fatigue, worry, excessive eating, dissatisfaction, climatic changes as well as purely Chinese healing factors such as blood stasis and stagnation of liver-qi.

To some it may seem strange that constipation can be a factor in brain and nervous disorders. But Chinese studies have found great success with stroke patient recovery—as high as 88 percent—simply by treating constipation naturally. Research is ongoing as to the effects of chinese medicine on strokes. Two doctors currently involved with stroke studies state, "Chinese medicine is of significance not only in preventing the occurrence of (stroke) but also in treating it" (Keji, 204-10).

Constipation leads to a toxic colon which can overburden the liver so that it is unable to filter out toxins effectively. Simply said, this can lead to brain and nervous system disorders. It is obvious then that a healthy colon is essential to an overall good state of health.

Preventing Autointoxication

• Learn to relax.
• Get plenty of sleep.
• Feed the body only nutritious foods.
• Exercise.
• Follow a cleansing program.
• Use colon, liver and blood formulas to clean, loosen, rebuild and neutralize toxins in the blood.

Dietary Guidelines

• Eat foods that offer nutritional support to the body.
• Add more vegetables, fruits and whole grain products to the diet.

• Avoid foods that cause stress on the body such as alcohol, tobacco, caffeine, sugar products and refined foods.

Nutritional Supplements

Calcium/Magnesium: This combination is excellent for the nervous system and body functions. These minerals help improve the health of the digestive tract, strengthen the nervous system, regulate heartbeat, and strengthen the muscular system. Minerals are necessary for enzyme function.

Vitamin/Mineral Supplement with Antioxidants: A good vitamin and mineral supplement will help to support the immune system and all body functions.

B-complex Vitamins with extra B12 and B6: The B vitamins the body cope with stress as well as help with the digestion process.

Vitamin C with Bioflavonoids: Vitamin C and bioflavonoids help with immune function, rid the body of toxins, encourage healing and prevent infections.

Herbal Supplements

Bee Pollen: This supplement helps to provide nutrients and restore vitality. It builds energy, nerves and the glandular system to promote a feeling of well-being.

Black Cohosh: This herb relaxes and builds the nervous system, calming and relieving pain.

Burdock: Burdock rids the liver of toxins that can interfere with a healthy nervous system. It aids with cleaning the glands, stomach, colon and in rebuilding the nervous system.

Capsicum: Capsicum helps restore the stomach and intestines with its stimulating action. It helps to improve absorption of other herbs and slowing fat absorption.

Ginger: Ginger is calming and soothing to the stomach. It also helps to stimulate and relax the nerves. Its naturally stimulating antibiotic properties help with cramps, nausea and in digesting other herbs.

Ginkgo: Ginkgo is a stimulant and alterative to restore memory and arterial blood flow to the nerves, brain. It also helps with depression, senility and vertigo.

Ginseng: Ginseng is a stimulant and tonic for the whole body. It is good for depression and fatigue.

Gotu Kola: This herb helps to stimulate brain function and memory. It also helps to relieve depression.

Kava: Kava helps to relax the muscles and as as a natural sedative to help with insomnia and nervous disorders.

Lady's Slipper: Lady's slipper is a tonic for an exhausted nervous system. It helps to calm and relax the nerves and brain.

Licorice: Licorice helps strengthen the adrenal glands, clean the liver and helps the body produce interferon to protect the immune system.

Oatstraw: This herb is excellent for all nervous disorders. It helps with insomnia, depression, fatigue, and nourishes the entire body.

Passionflower: Passionflower is soothing and relaxing for the nerves. It is useful for insomnia, fatigue, spasms and nervous tension.

Prickly Ash: This is a stimulant to aid in distributing herbs where they are needed. It helps repair nerves, relieves pain and increases immune function.

Skullcap: Skullcap relaxes and builds after nervous exhaustion. It is excellent for all nervous disorders.

Wood Betony: This herb helps to relieve pain, acts as a sedative, helps fatigue, enhances brain function and acts as a general tonic.

III. CANDIDIASIS

The overgrowth of the yeast organism *Candida albicans* is known as candidiasis. Candida is a normally occurring fungus that lives in the mucous membranes of the body, especially in the digestive tract and vagina. It can also be found in the sinuses, ear canals, and genitourinary tract. Under normal conditions the yeasts live in harmony with other organisms in the intestinal flora .The problem occurs when the unfriendly organisms proliferate to the point where they are detrimental to health. It is a more common condition in women of child-bearing years, though it can even infect infants and children. Some infants develop thrush, a form of candidiasis.

Problems arise when the body's natural immune function is weak due to various conditions such as lack of sleep, poor diet, stress, drugs, antibiotics, birth control pills, lack of exercise and environmental pollutants. Anything that weakens the immune system will in turn encourage the growth of candida. A strong and healthy immune system will contain the organisms, and they will only thrive when the host's resistance is low.

Microorganisms in the body are in constant competition for nourishment. When our systems are healthy and properly maintained, these life forms live in a harmonious balance. Our skin, intestinal tract, and mucous membranes all provide the perfect habitat for these bacteria and fungi. Through the release of certain toxins, they provide population control for each other. Developing a yeast infection can be the first sign that we are not in good health.

Candida multiplies and develops toxins which circulate in the bloodstream and lead to many symptoms, diseases, and chemical sensitivities in the body. Candida proliferation will often lead to a sensitivity to other molds and yeasts. Candida can produce a type of false estrogen so production of the true hormone is consequently inhibited. Similar phenomena can occur with the thyroid gland, resulting in menstrual irregularities and hypothyroid problems.

An additional detriment of candida overgrowth is that it produces an alcohol called ethanol. Ethanol grows rapidly when yeast has a food source, such as sugar. In severe cases more ethanol is produced than the liver can oxidize and eliminate. Acetaldehyde is another by-product of candida. It is related to formaldehyde and causes a variety of malfunctions in the body. It can also disrupt collagen production, fatty-acid oxidation and normal nerve function.

Causes of Candidiasis

Candida can flourish for a number of reasons, all involving a weakened immune system. The overuse of antibiotics is a serious concern and may be a major factor. Not only the bad bacteria are destroyed by antibiotics; friendly bacteria, a crucial part of the intestinal flora, also die when exposed to antibiotics. Because of this, the intestinal tract and other areas of the body are left vulnerable to yeast and other infections. When using antibiotics for an extended period of time or taking high doses, yeast infections may frequently occur. Antibiotics are often prescribed even when the infection is viral; this does nothing to "kill" the virus and only ends up destroying our body's helpful bacteria. The misuse of antibiotics is a major problem. Be aware that taking antibiotics orally is not the only problem. They are often given to cattle and chickens, thus appearing in meat and dairy products.

Candida also thrives on a high sugar diet, so a poor diet contributes greatly to a compromised immune system. Faulty nutrition may be the number one contributor to the development of a yeast infection. The human body was not designed to process large quantities of sugar. Refined sugar and carbohydrates impair the immune system by inhibiting the ability to assimilate nutrients. Sugar also plays a part in changing the character of the intestinal flora and providing the perfect habitat for yeasts to multiply.

Repeated pregnancies, nutritional deficiencies, birth control pills, steroid hormones and many different drugs are other things that can put a strain on the body and cause imbalances. The immune system is weakened, thus encouraging a candida-friendly environment. When the immune system is compromised for any one of a number of reasons, it leaves the body more vulnerable to conditions such as candida. If the defense mechanism in the body is inhibited, infectious organisms can invade and begin to reproduce.

The overgrowth of candida will not occur overnight. The immune system does not drop significantly in a short period of time. Weakening of the immune system will occur over a period of time due to a number of factors listed above. If you are aware of your body and what it need to maintain a state of health, candida should not be a problem for you.

If you do experience candidiasis, do not give up and resort to pharmaceutical drugs. In order for the body to heal after an overgrowth of candida has occurred, dietary changes must be made. It can be that simple a solution. It is also important to learn to control stress, reduce anxiety and get adequate rest. By far, the most effective approach is prevention. Nutritional therapies are the best approach.

Symptoms of Candidiasis

- fatigue
- bad breath
- sore throat
- chronic infections

- thyroid problems
- migraine headaches
- digestive disorders
- depression
- feeling disoriented

- panic attacks
- swollen glands
- constipation
- indigestion

Dietary Guidelines

- Eliminate sugar, honey, white flour products, yeast breads, wine, beer, fruit juices, cheese, mushrooms, junk food, refined foods, vinegar products and limit fruit to small amounts until the yeast is under control. Yeast multiples rapidly when starches and sugars are consumed regularly.
- Millet, brown rice and whole grains and vegetables are beneficial.
- Beans are a good source of protein.
- Almonds and nuts are good, but avoid peanuts.
- A great juice drink can be made from carrots, parsley, garlic and ginger.
- Add fiber to the diet—it helps clean the colon and eliminate toxins.

Nutritional Supplements

Acidophilus: Acidophilus is important for increasing friendly bacteria and in digestion. It also helps to prevent constipation and retard the growth of yeast organisms. It is best to take first thing in the morning before eating or just before bed.

Caprylic Acid: This naturally occurring essential fatty acids help to strengthen the immune system. It also helps to kill fungi and is easily absorbed in the intestinal tract.

Chlorophyll and Blue-Green Algae: These will help to purify the blood and provide essential nutrients. They also help the body produce its own interferon.

Olive Oil: Olive oil can be used on salads to help balance hormone levels and promote sugar metabolism.

Digestive Enzymes: Enzymes help to improve digestion and break down protein which can remain in the colon.

Germanium and Coenzyme Q-10: Germanium and coQ-10 help improve oxygen supply to the arteries.

Multi-Vitamin and Mineral Supplement: This will help to build the immune system and support the body. Chelated forms may be easier for the body to absorb.

Vitamin A and Beta Carotene: Vitamin A helps to stimulate the immune system and heal the mucous membranes. Beta carotene may be easier for the body to assimilate.

B-complex Vitamins: Yeast-free B vitamins are necessary for proper digestion and the absorption of nutrients. They also help the liver in eliminating toxins from the body.

Vitamin C with Bioflavonoids: Vitamin C and bioflavonoids help with immune function, rid the body of toxins, encourage healing and prevent infections.

Vitamin E: This antioxidant is helpful for strengthening the cardiovascular system and immune function.

Herbal Supplements

Barberry: Barberry can be used to treat conditions of yeast infections and to aid in their prevention. It also contains immune stimulating properties.

Cat's Claw: Cat's claw is found in the Peruvian rain forest and helps combat candidiasis throughout the entire intestinal tract.

Dong Quai: Dong quai helps to balance female hormones and nourish the female glands.

Echinacea: Echinacea is a natural antibiotic and helps to clean the lymphatic system.

Garlic: Garlic is a natural antibiotic. It also contains anti-fungal properties to help prevent and improve yeast infections.

Pau d'Arco: Pau d'arco is recommended to stimulate immune function and prevent disease. It contains powerful antibiotic, anti-fungal and anti-viral properties. It is recommended for healing infections.

IV. ENVIRONMENTAL POLLUTANTS

Each day we are bombarded by pollutants from our environment. The food we eat is full of pesticides, herbicides, preservatives, food additives, food coloring, nitrites and nitrates. Drinking water contains chlorine and metals including lead and cadmium. Pollutants in the air can cause many deadly diseases including cancer and lung ailments. Since there is no way to avoid contact with environmental pollutant entirely, it is important to aid the body in dealing with the problem.

Food Additives

Most people are concerned about the safety of the food they eat. Food additives, such as food coloring, preservatives, and pesticides, are all potentially harmful. There is evidence to support the belief that these additives are detrimental to the body. Natural, whole foods are believed superior because of the concentration of compounds in their natural state. The body more easily assimilates natural nutrients without additives. Food additives are usually included in food products to preserve freshness, increase flavor and add color. But even though the additives in use are approved by the government for consumption, they are not all safe. In his book *Healing With Whole Foods,* health expert Michael T. Murray comments on food additives, stating,

> The FDA has approved the use of over 2,800 different food additives. In 1985 the per capita daily consumption of these food additives was approximately 13 to 15 g. This astounding figure leads to many questions. Which food additives are safe? Which should be avoided? An extremist might argue that no food additive is safe. However, many food additives do fulfill important functions in our modern food supply. Many compounds approved as additives are natural in origin and possess health-promoting properties; others are synthetic compounds with known cancer-causing effects. Obviously, the most sensible approach is to focus on whole, natural foods and to avoid foods that are highly processed.

Food colorings are often added to foods, probably more so than anyone suspects. Not only are foods treated with coloring but with medications and vitamins are as well. These pose a serious threat for some individuals who are susceptible to allergic reactions. Exposure over a period of time can also increase allergic response. Some children are highly affected by food colorings.

Some commonly used preservatives include nitrates, nitrites, sulfites and sodium benzoate. They are added to lengthen the shelf-life and preserve freshness. But they can also cause problems for susceptible individuals. Natural, whole foods are preferred. Avoid processed foods that contain preservatives. They can cause allergic reactions and a link is suspected with some such as nitrates and nitrites to an increased risk of cancer.

Pesticides and herbicides are used to increase quality and crop production. But it is questionable whether the risks outweigh the advantages. Michael Murray suggests that there is a connection between exposure to toxins. Some health risks of longterm exposure to pesticides include cancer, birth defects, tremors, convulsions and nerve damage. Studies have found that farmers exposed to high doses of pesticides and herbicides are at a higher risk of developing certain types of cancer, even though they are thought to follow a relatively healthy lifestyle. Eat organically grown produce whenever possible. Many local grocers are carrying organic produce, and the extra cost is worth the health benefits.

Drinking Water

Everyone knows that water is necessary for life. But many individuals are concerned about the safety of our local water supplies. Chlorine and fluoride are often added, but there is also concern as to the toxic elements that find their way into the water—pesticides, herbicides, and some heavy metals. Water filters or bottled water may help to avoid the contaminants. There are many different systems available.

Fluoride in the drinking water may damage the body's ability to repair and rejuvenate. It can cause the breakdown of collagen, the protein that binds the body together. Dr. John Yiamouyiannis, in his book *Fluoride and the Aging Factor* says,

> Our immune system is the body's defense mechanism against bacteria, infections, viruses, and foreign proteins that get into our bloodstream. It attacks and destroys them. Fluoride interferes with the body's ability to reach and destroy the target. It reduces by 70 percent the ability of these white blood cells to reach the target. (26)

Chlorine can also cause problems. The standards for chlorine use in water are set for adults. This could leave children vulnerable to allergic reactions or other problems related to excessive amounts of chlorine. Some water supplies may contain extremely high levels of chlorine.

Air Pollution

There are several air pollutants that can cause serious afflictions like cancer, asthma or other lung ailments. Every year at least 100,000 deaths in the United States are attributed to air pollution. The EPA currently requires that states monitor for only six air contaminants including lead, ozone, carbon monoxide, nitrogen oxides, sulfur oxides and fine particulates (PM10). Some states monitor for other environmental pollutants. And new clean air legislation may mandate regulation and monitoring of other toxic air pollutants.

PM10 can cause and worsen respiratory illnesses including asthma, bronchitis, and pneumonia. PM10 suppresses the body's immune system and may even cause cancer. Carbon monoxide binds with hemoglobin in the bloodstream to decrease the ability of the blood in transporting oxygen and can result in dizziness, light-headedness, headaches and a slowing of reflexes. Recent research indicates that prolonged exposure to carbon monoxide can cause arterial and heart disease.

Lead is a very dangerous pollutant. It can affect blood forming tissue, the reproductive and nervous systems and the kidneys. Lead poisoning is also associated with neurological tissue damage and diminished learning potential, especially in children.

Toxins that are inhaled are assimilated 20 times faster than toxins that are eaten. When food is eaten and digested, hydrochloric acid helps to destroy toxins, germs, viruses, bacteria, parasites and worms.

Other Pollutants

Dioxin is a very potent synthetic chemical toxin. It is produced during the chlorine bleaching process. Wood pulp fiber is bleached with dioxin and used to make many everyday products such as toilet paper, sanitary napkins, tampons, paper towels, tissue, milk cartons, juice cartons, coffee filters, tea bags, paper plates and cups and the packaging for many processed foods.

Dioxin is also found in the environment, air and water. It is suspected of being an immune suppressant, causing liver disorders, cancer and birth defects. Toxic shock syndrome may be related to dioxin bleaching of tampons. The bleaching process sensitizes the vagina, leaving it vulnerable to infection. If the immune system is low, toxic shock syndrome could develop.

Environmental poisoning may be the cause of such diseases as Alzheimer's disease, lupus, multiple sclerosis, allergies and Lou Gehrig's disease. The leading causes of death in the United States include coronary heart disease, cancer and diabetes. These were all nonexistent or extremely rare before the Industrial Revolution. These diseases may be related to a slow poisoning from the polluted environment. Pesticides in the food, heavy metals in the air, inorganic minerals, and chlorine in the water may lead to chronic conditions.

Many believe that as a nation we are living longer and healthier lives. It has been based on the idea that the average life expectancy has increased over the last century. The fact is, the average life expectancy is higher, but most attribute this to a lower infant mortality rate. There has been an increase in heart disease, high blood pressure, cancer, degenerative diseases and autoimmune diseases. Simply said, those who live longer are not necessarily healthier nor happier.

Dietary Guidelines

- Cruciferous vegetable contain powerful antioxidants and nutrients that help protect against environmental toxins, balance hormones, and strengthen the immune system.
- Wheat grass juice, barley juice, green kamut and blue-green algae all help to protect the body from environmental toxins, strengthen the immune system, and nourish the blood.
- Eat less meat.
- Eat more whole grains, fresh fruit and vegetables and natural foods.
- Buy organic produce if possible.

Nutritional Supplements

Amino Acids: Amino acids are essential for healing and building the body. Methionine, glutathione, cysteine, glutamic acid and glycine are rich in sulfur, which helps the body defend itself against radiation, pollution, and in strengthening the entire body.

Antioxidants: Antioxidants are essential in combating environmental pollutants. The help strengthen the immune system.

Digestive Enzymes: These are necessary to ensure proper digestion and assimilation of nutrients. They help to clean undigested protein, germs, viruses, and parasites on a cellular level.

Selenium: Selenium is an antioxidant that stimulates immune function, prevents free radical damage and encourages healing.

Vitamin A: Vitamin A helps promote immune system function and aids in fighting free radical damage, which can occur from environmental pollutants.

Beta Carotene: Beta carotene is a water-soluble form of vitamin A which helps to strengthen the immune system.

B-Complex Vitamins: The B vitamins help to improve nervous system function and digestion. They are protective and strengthening for the nervous system.

Vitamin C with Bioflavonoids: Vitamin C is an antioxidant that helps to fight free radical damage and stimulate the immune function. It also aids in healing the body and removing toxins.

Vitamin E: Vitamin E aids in immune function, promotes healing and helps to prevent scarring.

Zinc: Zinc helps to protect the liver from toxins. It is also a strong immune stimulant.

Herbal Supplements

Burdock: Burdock is another excellent blood cleanser. It aids in neutralizing toxins in the blood and prevents the accumulation of toxins in the joints.

Cayenne: Cayenne is a stimulating herb often found in combinations to help improve their effectiveness. It contains antibacterial properties. It is also a tonic for the heart and strengthens the digestive and circulatory systems.

Comfrey Root: Comfrey contains healing properties and helps to rebuild the tissues in the lungs, stomach and digestive tract. It is a blood tonic. Comfrey helps to heal bones, cartilage, tendons and muscles. It is specific for healing asthmatic, lung and bronchial inflammation.

Fenugreek Seeds: Fenugreek is soothing for the mucous membranes. It helps to dissolve hard mucus and eliminate phlegm. It also dissolves fatty deposits and soothes and heals the digestive tract.

Garlic: Garlic contains sulfur, which binds with and deactivates radioactive isotopes, heavy metals such as cadmium, lead and mercury. It helps to lower high blood pressure and blood cholesterol levels. It aids in the prevention of blood clots. It also contains natural antibiotic properties to fight germs, bacteria and viruses.

Hyssop: Hyssop contains antispasmodic properties. It relaxes the nervous system, stimulates the liver to eliminate congestion and cleanses the lung from mucus.

Licorice: Licorice is healing for the digestive tract. It is a blood cleanser and helps to regulate hormone levels. It also helps strengthen the immune system and stimulate interferon production.

Lobelia: This herb aids in removing obstructions from the respiratory passages. It relaxes and cleans the lungs.

Marshmallow Root: Marshmallow root is healing for the mucous membranes and nourishing for the lungs, kidneys and colon.

Pau d'Arco: This is an herb to help cleanse the blood. It works to strengthen the immune system. It also helps contains natural antibiotic, antiviral, and antifungal properties.

V. HIATAL HERNIA

The hiatus is a small hole in the diaphragm through which the esophagus passes to join the stomach. The term hernia refers to a weakened area of muscle or a severely stretched muscle. A hiatal hernia occurs when for some reason the hole in the diaphragm weakens and enlarges, allowing a portion of the stomach to protrude upward through the hole beside the esophagus.

There are three types of hiatal hernia based on their severity, but the sliding hiatal hernia is the most common. A small part of the stomach slides back and forth in and out of the chest cavity through the small hole in the diaphragm. This type causes no problems and rarely any symptoms. Most people don't even know they have the disorder even though it is estimated to be present in up to 60 percent of the population by age sixty. Symptoms include chronic heartburn and belching.

Why hiatal hernias happens is not certain, but many natural health advocates feel there is a strong correlation between the incidence of hiatal hernia and diet. A high-fat diet will slow digestion and may cause irritation to the hiatal hernia. Obesity can also be an important factor. Obviously, it takes time for the body to heal, but a change in diet, an increase in exercise and a reduction in stress can help will help speed the process. Eating small meals in a calm place and chewing thoroughly will also reduced symptoms. A chiropractor may be helpful in manipulating the hiatal hernia back into place.

Causes of Hiatal Hernia

The medical community recognizes that the cause of hiatal hernia is difficult to determine. It is more common among obese individuals, middle-aged women and pregnant women. Some believe the condition is due to a congenital abnormality or a trauma to the hiatal area. A hiatal hernia often occurs when there is an increase in intra-abdominal pressure. This could be due to pressure created by straining to move hard feces when constipated.

Symptoms of Hiatal Hernia

Symptoms of hiatal hernia center around chronic heartburn and belching. Stomach acid sometimes come up into the throat which can cause burning and discomfort in the chest and throat. The tissue in the esophagus can become sore and irritated from the acid. Symptoms include the following:

- belching
- bloating
- regurgitation
- vomiting
- constipation
- burning in upper chest
- pressure below breastbone
- heartburn
- intestinal gas
- nausea
- diarrhea
- fatigue
- allergies
- dizziness

Dietary Guidelines

- Drink large glasses of water throughout the day.
- Eat in a calm environment.
- Eat several small meals daily.
- Eat a high-fiber diet. (see Chapter Four on fiber)
- Add more grains to the diet.
- Eat more fruit, vegetables and natural foods.
- Eat less meat.
- Avoid fatty and fried foods.
- Avoid coffee, tea, alcohol, cola drinks and smoking.
- Do not eat within two hours of bedtime.

Nutritional Supplements

Antioxidants: Antioxidants will help to strengthen the immune system and heal the mucous membranes of the digestive system.

Chlorophyll: Chlorophyll is nourishing and helps the body heal the esophagus and stomach.

Coenzyeme Q-10: This supplement can help by providing oxygen to the cells to promote healing and increase strength.

Minerals: Minerals are needed to help heal and balance the body.

Papaya Enzyme: Papaya can help encourage good digestion and healing.

Vitamin A: Vitamin A helps to fight excess acid accumulation and to enhance the immune system.

B-Complex Vitamins: The B-complex vitamins are necessary for digestion. They are needed to help the enzymes function.

Vitamin C: Vitamin C is helpful for the immune system and in healing tissue.

Zinc: Zinc helps repair damaged tissue.

Herbal Supplements

Aloe Vera: Aloe vera helps to promote healing of the digestive tract.

Gentian: Gentian helps to heal the stomach and improves weak muscular tone of the digestive tract.

Ginger: This is a well-known herb that helps with the digestive system. It helps improve digestion, fight indigestion and relieve nausea and an upset stomach.

Goldenseal: Goldenseal nourishes the digestive tract and improves digestion. It can help heal mucous membranes in the digestive system.

Marshmallow Root: Marshmallow is soothing and healing for the digestive tract. It helps with gastrointestinal disorders.

Slippery Elm: This herb helps to neutralize stomach acidity and absorbs gas. It aids in the digestion of milk. Slippery elm also helps reduce inflammation and irritations of the mucous membranes.

VI. ILEOCECAL VALVE SYNDROME

The ileocecal valve is located at the point where the small intestine opens into the ascending colon. It is comprised of sphincter muscles which serve to close the ileum (the third and lowest division of the small intestine). In this way the ileocecal valve helps to keep the digesting material in the small intestine until the food has been changed by the digestive juices and absorbed. It also functions to prevent a reflux of material from the colon back into the small intestine.

The valve passes the mixture of unusable food residue, mucus, bile and other excretions from the small intestine into the colon in small successive doses. This prevents an overload of material for the body to eliminate. Dr. John Harvey Kellogg, M.D., a colon specialist at the turn of the century, says in his book *Colon Hygiene:*

> One of the consequences of chronic constipation is incompetency of the ileocecal valve. By over-distention, the intestine becomes so widely dilated that the lips of the valve no longer come in contact and so its check valve action is prevented, and the putrefying contents of the colon readily pass backward into the small intestine. When the ileocecal valve is incompetent, it is, of course, incompetent to gases as well as liquids. Incompetency of the ileocecal valve is both a consequence and a cause of constipation. The valve is often rendered incompetent by over-stretching of the bowel, usually the result of obstruction in the descending or pelvic colon. When once the valve is crippled, the constipation is made worse by the loss of check valve action, which aids the forward movement of the bowel contents, so that the food residues oscillate back and forth between the large and the small bowel. The stagnation resulting from this condition readily leads to infection of the cecum and appendicitis, and to more remote affections, through extension of the infection backward along the small

intestine to the duodenum, stomach, gallbladder, liver and pancreas, causing inflammation of the gall ducts and gallbladder, gallstones, pancreatitis and possible diabetes, duodenal and gastric ulcers, and various other allied affections. (141)

Ileocecal valve disorder could be one cause of chronic conditions. The toxic material of the colon can enter back into the small intestine and rapidly be reabsorbed. This allows for various toxins to reenter the body, which may lead to disease.

At a symposium held at the Royal Medical Society of Great Britain in 1918, sixty doctors presented their views on autointoxication and intestinal toxemia. The competency of the ileocecal valve was widely discussed. Dr. James T. Case and Dr. W. Curtis Brigham, D.O. Chief of Staff and colon specialist at the Monte-Sano Hospital, routinely found that many diseases were caused by the incompetency of the ileocecal valve. Dr. Brigham detected many dysfunctional ileocecal valves by X-ray examination after a barium meal. While performing surgery he removed adhesions in the gastrointestinal tract and repaired the ileocecal valve. Dr. Brigham discovered that these poisons were the cause of many cases of epileptiform seizures. By eliminating the problem, he cleared up as many as fifty percent of his epilepsy cases (Rodifer, 21).

Ileocecal Valve Syndrome and Parasites

The prevalence of parasites in the body is often overlooked by medical professionals, but some believe that parasite infestation can lead to ileocecal valve syndrome. Irritation or inflammation caused by the parasites can somehow cause the valve to remain open or to close only partially. When the valve remains open, toxins can be reabsorbed in the bloodstream. The condition will persist until an individual undergoes a parasite cleanse to rid the body of the invaders.

Causes of Ileocecal Valve Syndrome

Some natural health professionals feel that iliocecal valve syndrome affects up to fifty percent of the population. The reasons for the ileocecal valve to remain open are not entirely understood, but may be due in part to poor eating habits, parasites or a lack of fiber in the diet.

Symptoms of Ileocecal Valve Syndrome

- constipation/diarrhea
- irregular bowel movements
- lower right bowel tenderness
- immune weakness
- duodenal ulcers
- fatigue
- acne
- migraines

Dietary Guidelines

- Eat a diet high in fiber, including whole grains. Soak the grains and cook to avoid irritating the valve.
- Avoid constipating food, such as dairy, meat, bananas, etc.
- Eat stewed prunes, figs and raisins for breakfast.
- Add more fresh fruits and vegetables to the diet. The softer raw vegetables such as leaf lettuce, spinach, avocados, sprouts and tomatoes should be used at first.
- Reduce the amount of meat eaten.
- Take a fiber supplement to avoid constipation.
- Implementing a juice fast two to three days a week will help to speed the healing process of the digestive tract.
- Thermos-cooked grains are healing to the digestive tract. They are rich in enzymes, vitamins, minerals and protein. This slow-cook process prevents destruction of the vital enzymes.
- Millet, buckwheat and basmati brown rice can be eaten for breakfast. They are easy to digest and very nourishing.

- Raw vegetables and fruits, steamed vegetables, yams and avocados are all helpful in healing the digestive tract.

Nutritional Supplements

Acidophilus: Acidophilus helps to destroy putrefactive bacteria in the intestinal tract. Putrefactive bacteria liberates histamine, a toxic substance that is the result of undigested protein. Vitamin K and B-complex vitamins can be synthesized in the small intestine when acidophilus is present.

Antioxidants: Vitamins A, C, E, selenium and zinc are antioxidants that support the immune system. They help the body in healing and preventing infection

Blue-Green Algae and Chlorophyll: These supplements are cleansing and healing to the digestive tract and the blood.

Calcium/Magnesium: These minerals help improve the health of the digestive tract. They help to strengthen the nervous system, regulate heartbeat, and strengthen the muscular system. Minerals are necessary for enzyme function.

Essential Fatty Acids (flaxseed oil, salmon oil, evening primrose oil, borage oil and black currant oil): Essential fatty acids are need for a healthy glandular system. They help to regulate hormone function.

Plant Digestive Enzymes: These help digest food when it is eaten. When they are taken between meals, they help break down the protein in the blood and cells so the body can eliminate toxins.

Vitamin A (Beta carotene): This vitamin is necessary for tissue repair and strengthening the immune system.

B-Complex Vitamins: The B vitamins are essential for intestinal health. They help strengthen the nervous system and also are essential to the digestion process.

Vitamin C with Bioflavonoids: These are necessary for the adrenal and thyroid glands to supply essential hormones.

Along with calcium, they also help improve collagen supplies and contribute to digestive tract health.

Herbal Supplements

Aloe Vera Juice: Aloe vera juice helps to heal and repair tissue in the digestive tract.

Cat's Claw: Cat's claw is an herb with anti-inflammatory properties that enhances the immune system. It helps to strip the colon walls of accumulated waste and promote intestinal healing.

Comfrey: Comfrey helps with digestion by promoting the production of pepsin. It is healing and strengthening on the body.

Goldenseal: Goldenseal helps soothe and heal the digestive system. It also improves digestion.

Grape Seed Extract: The proanthocyanidins in grape seed extract have impressive antioxidant properties. They help to reduce inflammation and promote healing.

Licorice: Licorice is soothing on the digestive tract and has been used to prevent and treat ulcers. It works as a laxative and reduces inflammation of the digestive system.

Pau d'Arco: This herb helps promote healing and fights disease.

Slippery Elm: Slippery elm is healing to the mucous membranes. It buffers the effects of irritations and inflammations of the mucous membranes.

VII. Leaky Gut Syndrome

A syndrome is a group of signs and symptoms that collectively characterize or indicate a particular disease or abnormal condition. One disease may have many different symptoms to distinguish it from other conditions. Some syndromes are closely related and an individual may suffer from more than one at a time. Leaky gut syndrome is one condition that can lead to and may be associated with other serious disorders.

The gastrointestinal tract is designed to perform many important and essential functions for the body. It digests and assimilates nutrients for use in the body. Vitamins and minerals attach to proteins to cross the gut lining and enter the bloodstream. The gastrointestinal tract also works to detoxify chemicals and harmful substances that enter the body and fight infection. If the gastrointestinal tract is compromised for various reasons, the body can suffer serious consequences.

Dr. Sherry A. Rogers, M.D., explains leaky gut syndrome. "The leaky gut syndrome is a poorly recognized but extremely common problem that is seldom tested for. It represents a hyperpermeable intestinal lining. In other words, large spaces develop between the cells of the gut wall and bacteria, toxins and food leak in" (34-35).

If the lining of the intestinal tract becomes more permeable than normal, it can lead to serious health concerns. The large spaces that develop between the cells of the gut wall allow toxic material to enter the bloodstream. Under normal conditions these toxic substances would be eliminated, but when leaky gut syndrome occurs, parasites, bacteria, fungi, toxins, fats and other foreign matter not normally absorbed enter the bloodstream. These microbes can put an enormous strain on the liver and lessen its ability to detoxify.

The enlarged spaces in the gut wall also allow for the entrance of larger-than-normal protein molecules. These proteins are not completely broken down so the immune system recognizes them as foreign matter and makes antibodies to fight them. When these antibodies are produced, the body begins to recognize relatively common foods or other substances as detrimental and this leads to allergic reactions. An inflammatory response may occur when the food or substance is next consumed. If the inflammation occurs in a joint, rheumatoid arthritis may result. If the antibodies attack the gut lining, various gastrointestinal problems can develop, such as Crohn's disease or colitis. Some cases of asthma are thought to be related to leaky gut syndrome because the inflammatory condition that arises after ingesting a certain food triggers the asthma. Other associated problems include migraines, eczema, and immune problems. It is easy to see how this antibody response can produce symptoms in just about any organ or area of the body.

The leaky gut syndrome is a common health condition primarily due to today's lifestyle, but many times the problem is overlooked by medical professionals. The symptoms may be masked for a time but the underlying cause remains.

Causes of Leaky Gut Syndrome

The overuse and misuse of antibiotics is considered a major cause of leaky gut syndrome. Broad spectrum antibiotics can kill all the friendly as well as the bad bacteria in the intestinal tract. This can lower the capacity to fight fungus such as *Candida albicans* and *Clostridia difficle* that are often associated with colitis. Antibiotics can also kill the bacteria that break down complex foods and synthesize essential vitamins. The friendly bacteria help to fight infection and defend the body to keep parasites and fungi under control.

A poor diet high in carbohydrates, sugar, alcohol and caffeine can irritate the lining of the gut. This can cause inflammation leading to hyperpermeability (leaky gut syndrome).

A deficiency in enzymes can also lead to leaky gut syndrome. Enzymes help to break down, digest, and assimilate nutrients. Cooked and processed foods are depleted of essential enzymes. Raw foods such as fruits and vegetables contain enzymes. A poor diet lacking in enzymes can impair digestion and cause inflammation of the gut lining. If adequate amounts of enzymes are not available in the body, leaky gut syndrome may develop.

Non-steroidal anti-inflammatory drugs (NSAIDS) also contribute to leaky gut syndrome. Some NSAIDS include ibuprofen, ASA, indomethiacin, aspirin, and naproxen sodium. Problems occur as these drugs cause irritation and inflammation in the intestinal lining which in turn causes hyperpermeability between the cells.

Other contributors to the syndrome are chemicals, heavy metals, pesticides and other toxins that can damage the digestive tract. These foreign materials can cause inflammation and hyperpermeability between cells in the gut lining. Organisms such as *Giardia lamblia* or *Klebsiella citrobacter* can also compromise the gut lining and contribute to leaky gut syndrome.

Symptoms of Leaky Gut Syndrome

- frequent colds, infections
- fungal disease
- food intolerances/ allergies
- chemical sensitivities
- abdominal distention
- toxic feelings
- cognitive/memory deficits
- shortness of breath
- aches and pains
- nausea after eating
- diarrhea
- abdominal pain
- skin rashes
- difficulty exercising
- fatigue
- low-grade fever

Diseases Associated with Leaky Gut Syndrome

- IBS
- eczema
- food sensitivities
- liver disease
- asthma
- Lupus
- chronic fatigue syndrome

- acne
- psoriasis
- cystic fibrosis
- rheumatoid arthritis
- celiac disease
- fibromyalgia
- autism

Dietary Guidelines

The intestinal tract can be healed by adding more raw food to the diet, especially fresh vegetable juices. Fasting on vegetable juices will help to repair and provide enzymes necessary for health and digestion. A diet consisting of 60-70 percent raw food will help to reverse the degeneration that has occurred in the gut lining, as well as improve energy and vitality.

Cleansing the digestive tract and the colon will help assure that the body is digesting and assimilating essential nutrients for healing and restoring health. Avoid low-fiber foods, cooked foods, white flour products, sugar, fried foods and processed foods. Eat a diet rich in fiber, fruits and vegetables. Fiber formulas, blood cleansers and bowel formulas can help to clean toxins from the body that can lead to chronic disease. To obtain and maintain optimal health, try some of the following dietary suggestions.

- Regularly consume vegetable juice combinations, including carrot, celery, and endive; carrot, parsley, cabbage and garlic; ginger, parsley, garlic, carrots and celery juices.

- Fasting on these juices two to three days a week will help to speed the healing process of the digestive tract.
- Thermos-cooked grains are healing on the digestive tract. They are rich in enzymes, vitamins, minerals and protein. This slow-cook process prevents destruction of the vital enzymes.
- Drink plenty of liquids, including pure water, electrolyte drinks without added sugar, fruit juices diluted with pure water, and almond milk, which is rich in calcium, magnesium and protein. Almond milk can be added to fruit drinks.
- Millet, buckwheat and basmati brown rice can be eaten for breakfast. They are easy for the body to digest and very nourishing.
- Raw vegetables and fruits, steamed vegetables, yams and avocados are all helpful in healing the digestive tract.

Nutritional Supplements

Acidophilus: Acidophilus helps to destroy putrefactive bacteria in the intestinal tract. Putrefactive bacteria liberates histamine, a toxic substance that is the result of undigested protein. Vitamin K and B-complex vitamins can be synthesized in the small intestine when acidophilus is present.

Antioxidants: Vitamins A, C, E, selenium and zinc are antioxidants that support the immune system. They protect the cells from damage.

Blue-Green Algae and Chlorophyll: These are cleansing and healing to the digestive tract and the blood.

Calcium/Magnesium: These minerals help improve the health of the digestive tract. They aid in strengthening the nervous system, regulate heartbeat, and strengthen the muscular system. Minerals are necessary for enzyme function.

Essential Fatty Acids (flaxseed oil, salmon oil, evening primrose oil, borage oil and black currant oil): Essential fatty acids are need for a healthy glandular system. They help to regulate hormone function.

Plant Digestive Enzymes: These help digest food when it is eaten. When they are taken between meals, they help break down the protein in the blood and cells so the body can eliminate the toxins.

Vitamin A (Beta Carotene): This is vital for tissue repair and strengthening the immune system.

B-complex Vitamins: The B vitamins are essential for intestinal health. They help prevent depression, strengthen the nervous system, improve fatigue, reduce sugar cravings, prevent bloating and stabilize weight fluctuations. They also help to eliminate the "bad" estrogen from the liver.

Vitamin C with Bioflavonoids: These are necessary for the adrenal and thyroid glands to supply essential hormones. They also help improve collagen production.

Herbal Supplements

Aloe Vera Juice: Aloe vera juice helps to heal and repair tissue in the digestive tract.

Cat's Claw: Cat's claw is an immune enhancing herb with anti-inflammatory properties. It helps to strip the colon walls of accumulated waste and promote intestinal healing.

Comfrey: Comfrey helps with digestion by promoting the production of pepsin.

Goldenseal: Goldenseal helps soothe and heal the digestive system. It also improves digestion.

Grape Seed Extract: The proanthocyanidins in grape seed extract have impressive antioxidant properties. They help to reduce inflammation and promote healing.

Licorice: Licorice is soothing on the digestive tract and has been used to prevent and treat ulcers. It works as a laxative and reduces inflammation of the digestive system.

Pau d'Arco: This herb helps promote healing and fight disease.

Slippery Elm: Slippery elm is healing on the mucous membranes. It buffers against irritations and inflammations of the mucous membranes.

VIII. PARASITES AND WORMS

Parasites and worms are becoming a real problem in the United States. They are scavengers that live within, upon or at the expense of another organism—the host—without contributing to its survival. These parasites can reside in the gastrointestinal tract and feed on toxins and waste material in the body. The most common types include roundworms (hookworms, pinworms and threadworms) and tapeworms. The main problem is that the parasites expel waste material that can be extremely toxic to the host. Some parasites cause irritations to body tissue that may lead to an inflammatory response. Some may also rob the host of blood and nutrients.

Due to limited sanitation measures people often ingest contaminated food, water and dirt. The good news is that if the body is free of toxins and produces adequate amounts of hydrochloric acid, it can destroy parasites, worms and their larva. Anyone in a poor state of health is more susceptible to parasites. A diet rich in fat, starch and sugar provides food for parasites and worms.

Parasites and worms may be associated with a great many diseases—colon disorders, AIDS, some types of cancer, chronic fatigue syndrome, and candidiasis. Unfortunately, most medical professionals never check for the the possible presence of parasites and worms.

Causes of Parasites

Worms and parasites can be contracted in many different ways. An individual may unknowingly come in contact with waste material that is contaminated. Walking barefoot on contaminated soil can lead to infestation. Ingestion of larvae or eggs from handling meat or partially cooked meat is a problem. Pork is often contaminated with parasites, even when it is cooked. *Giardia lamblia* is often found in stream and lakes and is then introduced into drinking water supplies.

Along with actual contact with worms and parasites, frequent use of antibiotics, poor diet, other medications, and stress can reduce beneficial intestinal flora and provide an environment where parasites and worms will thrive.

Symptoms of Parasites

- poor absorption of nutrients
- abdominal pain
- diarrhea
- colon disorders
- growth problems in children
- diminished immune function
- colitis
- weight loss
- loss of appetite
- anemia
- rectal itching
- fatigue
- gas and bloating
- headaches

Dietary Guidelines

- Eat a high-fiber diet full of raw vegetables, fruits and whole grains.
- Pumpkin seeds, pomegranate seeds, sesame seeds and figs can help rid the body of parasites and worms.
- Garlic, onions, cabbage and carrots contain sulphur, which aids in expelling parasites from the body.
- Drink a lot of purified water.

- Avoid sugar, refined foods, white flour products, chocolate, alcohol, tobacco and caffeine.
- Limit or avoid entirely meat products, especially pork.
- If meat is eaten, make sure it is fully cooked.
- Hydrochloric acid and digestive enzymes are very important and supplements may be necessary. The hydrochloric acid helps to kill parasites when sufficient amount are available.
- Blood, colon and liver cleansers are necessary to get rid of the toxins that feed parasites and worms.

Nutritional Supplements

Acidophilus: Acidophilus is essential to help maintain and encourage normal intestinal flora.

Essential Fatty Acids: The essential fatty acids help to heal and protect the gastrointestinal tract.

Multivitamin/Mineral Supplement: A multivitamin and mineral supplement is essential to increase the immune function and help the body to recover.

B-Complex Vitamins: The B vitamins help to prevent anemia (B12), aid in digestion, detoxify the liver and help support the nervous system.

Vitamin C with Bioflavonoids: These help to prevent infection, increase immune function and promote healing in the body.

Zinc: Zinc helps to increase the immune function and encourage healing.

Herbal Supplements

Aloe Vera Juice: Aloe vera juice is healing and soothing on the digestive tract.

Black Walnut: Black walnut is effective in killing many parasites and worms.

Burdock: Burdock aids in cleansing the blood and in eliminating parasites from the body.

Echinacea: Echinacea is a natural antibiotic and encourages immune function. It also aids in killing parasites in the digestive tract.

Garlic: Garlic contains antibiotic and antiparasitic properties, helping to expel parasites from the body.

Goldenseal: Goldenseal is another effective natural antibiotic which helps to kill worms and parasites.

Grape Seed Extract: Grapeseed extract helps to kill parasites in the body.

Pumpkin Seeds: Pumpkin seeds are helpful in expelling worms.

CHAPTER FOUR

THE IMPORTANCE OF FIBER

Fiber is an important item that has come to the public's attention, thanks to the media and a growing mountain of medical data. Fiber has always been considered important in the natural health world, but was long neglected and not considered essential by most people involved in standard medicine. Finally, the medical community is beginning to realize something that natural health advocates have professed for years. The American Medical Association has joined the National Cancer Institute, the American Heart Association and the American Dietetic Association in encouraging the public to eat foods high in fiber, such as whole grains, legumes, fruits and vegetables. More attention is being placed on fiber and its importance, and this is one area in which the medical community and natural health field agree.

For decades, fiber was thought to have no nutritional benefits; so it was removed from foods to make them smooth and more appetizing. While the diets of many individuals still lack good sources of fiber, more and more people are realizing the healthy contribution fiber can make in their diets. In *The Complete Fiber Fact Book,* Rita Elkins states:

> Current data which is slowly emerging strongly suggests that we look at the value of whole foods very carefully. After all, our ancestors did not go to the cereal aisle and buy wheat germ or oat bran, they ate the whole grain as nature intended. When we eat bran or fragmented flours separately, our living systems react to them differently than when they are part of a whole, integrated food. When cereal grains, fruits, vegetables, beans, nuts and seeds are tampered with, altered or fragmented they have become artificial foods to some extent. (25)

Researchers have found fiber to be very important in protecting and preventing many detrimental conditions. It is this material that is important in keeping the digestive process moving and the intestinal system functioning efficiently. Fiber has been found to lower blood pressure, lower blood cholesterol levels, stabilize blood sugar levels, help protect against colon cancer, remove toxins from the body, prevent constipation, protect against hemorrhoids and promote weight control. Fiber is obviously an important element of a healthy diet!

I. THE STRUCTURE OF FIBER

Fiber is found in the cell walls of plants. Every plant cell has a wall of fiber and this is what works to keep the plant rigid. Fiber is usually considered the part of food that is not digestible. It consists of both water-insoluble fibers which absorb water, swell and add bulk, and water-soluble fibers. Some foods contain both types of fiber. The composition of fiber is determined by the species of plant, but the majority of plant cell walls are composed of approximately 35 percent insoluble fiber, 45 percent soluble fiber, 17 percent lignins, 3 percent proteins and 2 percent ash.

Insoluble fiber is primarily composed of cellulose and hemicellulose and is found in whole grains, fruits and vegetables. Cellulose is a portion of fiber that is nondigestible and found in the outer layer of vegetables, whole grains and fruits. Wheat bran is a form of insoluble fiber. It takes on water, increasing the size and weight of waste matter as it travels through the colon. This helps decrease transit time and increase the regularity of bowel movements. Insoluble fiber has been linked to aiding in the removal of toxins and excess hormones from the body, reducing constipation and promoting regular bowel movements, improving digestion and lowering the risk of bowel diseases and colon cancer.

Water-soluble fibers are found in apples, citrus fruits, oats, legumes, psyllium and some vegetables. They are known as gums, pectins, lignins and mucilages. When water-soluble fibers are digested, they form a gel-like substance that absorbs water in the intestinal tract. Increasing soluble fiber in the diet has been found to help prevent blood-sugar swings, lower cholesterol, decrease the risk of heart disease, and aid in controlling high blood pressure.

Bran refers to the fibrous covering surrounding whole grains. It the the portion of the fiber generally discarded during the milling process. Bran holds water very efficiently so it is a great bulking tool and can reduce transit time. As the use of bran is decreased, the incidence of many diseases is increased.

II. TYPES OF FIBER

Trying to decipher the scientific data regarding the best types of fiber to add to the diet can be distressing. There are seven basic forms of fiber, including the following:

Pectin: Pectin helps to slow down the absorption of food after eating, which is beneficial for individuals with diabetes. It is recommended for individuals suffering from hypoglycemia or diabetes because of its ability to cause a gradual rise in the blood glucose levels. It helps to remove toxins from the body, reduce the effects of radiation therapy, lower cholesterol levels, and reduce the risk of heart disease and gallstones. Good sources of pectin include carrots, beets, cabbage, citrus fruits, apples, grapes, bananas, dried peas, green beans and onion skin.

Cellulose: Cellulose is an insoluble source of fiber. It is an indigestible complex carbohydrate found in the outer fibrous covering of vegetables and fruits. This type of fiber helps with conditions such as varicose veins, colitis, constipation, and hemorrhoids. Good sources include wheat bran, beets, peas, broccoli, carrots, lima beans, Brazil nuts, pears, apples, whole grains and green beans.

Hemicellulose: This is another indigestible complex carbohydrate source of fiber. It is the matrix of the cell walls of the plants containing cellulose fibers. Bacteria in the bowels break down the fiber. Hemicellulose can hold a lot of water and can help with conditions such as weight loss, colon cancer, constipation, and toxin elimination. Sources include psyllium seeds, oat bran, apples, pears, bananas, beans, corn, cabbage, whole grains, peppers and green vegetables.

Lignin: Lignin is the non-carbohydrate cell wall material. Lignin fibers have been found to help lower cholesterol levels and prevent the formation of gallstones. It binds with bile acids removing them before they can form stones. It also can be changed by friendly bacteria in the intestines into a substance which can inhibit the action of the "bad" estrogen linked to breast cancer. It is recommended for individuals with diabetes, breast or colon cancer. Good sources of lignins include flaxseeds, wheat, potatoes, apples, cabbage, carrots, potatoes, peaches, tomatoes, strawberries, Brazil nuts, carrots, peas and green beans.

Gums: Gums are water-soluble sources of fiber that help to repair damaged areas. Most types of gums are taken from the stems or seeds of tropical or subtropical trees and shrubs. Gums tend to form a gel in the small intestine, helping to bind with toxins and acids and removing them from the body. They have been found to help reduce levels of cholesterol and triglycerides. Some sources are guar gum, gum arabic, flaxseed gum, locust seed gum, and psyllium seed gum.

Mucilages: Mucilages are removed from seeds and seaweeds and are often used as a thickening and stabilizing agent. They hold water and work as bulking agents. Sources include legumes, psyllium and guar.

III. TRANSIT TIME

After food enters the mouth, it gradually works its way through the body. The time it takes for the process to occur may have a great deal to do with the amount of fiber in the diet. Cultures who show excellent health levels are known to eat foods high in fiber and have a shorter digestion/transit time. *The Complete Fiber Fact Book* explains:

Western nations that eat diets low in fiber have longer transit times than third-world countries. It is commonplace for an American to have a transit time of three days to two weeks in cases of severe constipation. Eight to thirty-five hours is typically seen in cultures where whole grains, fruits and plants are routinely consumed. Normally, adults who eat from thirty-five to forty-five grams of fiber every day have an average transit time of approximately thirty-six to forty-eight hours. Transit time can vary from person to person, and if you're a woman, it can be 24 percent slower than for men. Changes in transit time from one day to the next are also common; however, it is not normal to have three bowel movements a day and then go without one for a week. (32)

Fiber helps to decrease the elimination time by speeding up the various digestion/excretion processes. It seems that the faster food is eliminated through the system, the greater the benefits. Fiber can keep toxins from building up in the colon by keeping the bowels moving. High-protein and -fat diets are absorbed mainly in the intestines. This may lead to constipation problems. With a high-fiber diet, cholesterol, fats and toxins are excreted from the body at a faster pace. The theory is that the less time toxins and carcinogenic substances remain in the bowels, the chances of them causing problems are greatly reduced. Diets low in dietary fiber allow the food to remain longer in the intestines, which causes toxins to build up the chances of invoking disease to rise. The fiber will not cure cancer, but it may help in preventing problems for susceptible individuals. With a high-fiber diet, the bowel wall will more likely remain strong and clean.

If waste material remains in the colon for a long period of time, putrefaction can occur. Toxic compounds may work their way into the bloodstream; if this occurs, we have to rely on the liver to filter them out. This is known as autointoxication. Some of the toxins can be extremely detrimental—

even carcinogenic in nature—and can lead to serious, chronic conditions. Longer transit time may also lead to hemorrhoids and diverticulitis because of the pressure and straining required. Chronic intestinal gas can also occur with increased transit time.

IV. FANTASTIC FIBER

Some studies have made fantastic claims as to the importance of fiber. Lower cholesterol levels have been attributed to fiber intake, as have the prevention of heart disease and colon cancer. The important thing to remember is that most people do not get enough fiber. The National Cancer Institute has recommended that people eat at least twenty to thirty-five grams of fiber each day. And many experts suggest as much as forty grams per day. The average American probably consumes only ten to fifteen grams of fiber per day.

In cultures where fruits, vegetables, and whole grains are eaten in abundance, there is less incidence of obesity, colitis, appendicitis, cancer and polyps of the colon. Experts attribute this to the high-fiber content found in the average diet. The best method of increasing fiber in *your* diet is to include whole grains, brown rice, oats, pasta,and ample amounts of fruits and vegetables. Be aware of what you are eating. Fast foods are not only high in fat, but very low in fiber. Fiber should be gradually introduced into the diet as to avoid intestinal problems such as diarrhea, bloating, and flatulence.

V. DISEASE AND THE FIBER CONNECTION

Appendicitis

Appendicitis is an acute inflammation of the appendix, which is a small branch off the intestine. Its function is not entirely known, though there has been some lymph tissue found which may have an important immune function of protecting the body from local infection. A blockage from waste material is thought to be a contributing factor in appendicitis. Some health professionals strongly believe that there is a connection between appendicitis and fiber consumption. Appendectomies are rarely performed in third world countries where high-fiber diets are consumed.

In *The Healing Foods,* Patricia Hausman and Judith Benn Hurley suggest how fiber can prevent appendicitis:

> Of all possible dietary explanations for appendicitis, a low-fiber intake has been suspected most. The case for a protective effect from fiber rests on facts such as these. Appendicitis tends to be more common in countries where the diet is low in fiber. During the war, when appendicitis rates fell, residents of Switzerland and the English Channel Islands were eating more fiber (and less fat) than usual. Surveys in African cities by Denis Burkitt, M.D., have shown that appendicitis is ten times more common in whites than in blacks. In Africa, of course, the former are more likely to follow a Western-type diet. Some research shows that children who develop appendicitis eat less fiber. Jean Brender, Ph.D., and associates at the University of Washington School of Public Health reported in 1985 that children who had eaten the diets richest in fiber were only half as likely to develop the disease. (35-36)

There are some health care professionals who do not believe in the fiber/appendicitis link, but it is certainly convincing when you look at the data from other nations. Appendectomies are the number one abdominal surgery performed in the Western world, but are quite rare in third-world countries. Appendectomies were also quite rare in the Western populations before the introduction of refined foods. Adding fiber to the diet and drinking plenty of water could be an important factor in the prevention of appendicitis. Keep the bowels moving by eating whole foods high in fiber.

Breast Cancer

Breast cancer is the most common cancer for women. The disease involves a malignant tumor in the breast tissue. If the condition continues, it may spread to other parts of the body. Breast cancer is rarely seen in Japan, where a low-fat, high-fiber diet is regularly eaten. It is easy to understand the correlation between colon cancer and a low-fiber diet, but many have difficulty with the concept of a low-fiber diet and a higher risk of breast cancer.

Why is this? Fiber may help protect against breast cancer in several ways. First, transit time is lessened, allowing for quicker removal of cancer-causing substances, one of which is estrogen. Jon J. Michnovicz, in his book *How To Reduce Your Risk of Breast Cancer,* suggests that many women are unaware of the amount of estrogen in their bowel movements. Estrogen finds its way into the intestines from the liver and needs to be eliminated. Waste can sit in the bowel for twenty-four hours or more, allowing for the estrogen to be reabsorbed into the body (114).

Hormones are essential for life but an overabundance of certain hormones circulating in the bloodstream has been linked to certain cancerous conditions. Fiber may help by eliminating hormones from the body, and certain types of fiber may be more effective than others. Wheat bran, an insoluble fiber, has been linked to lowering estrogen levels. Insoluble fiber binds with substances like estrogen and eliminates them through the bowels.

Cholesterol

Cholesterol is a wax-like substance which can accumulate in the arteries, often adhering to arterial walls near the heart. There are actually two types of cholesterol: low-density lipoproteins (LDL), which are considered "bad" cholesterol, and high-density lipoproteins (HDL), thought to be "good" cholesterol.

LDL cholesterol is the type which can cause serious damage to the artery walls. It contains a chemical known as apolipoprotein-B, which is responsible for the problem. The apolipoprotein-B adheres to arterial walls, resulting in plaque build-up, and inhibits the smooth flow of blood. When the adherence is near the heart, the individual is at risk of developing coronary heart disease. High LDL cholesterol levels have been linked to heart disease, which can lead to a heart attack or stroke.

HDL cholesterol is thought to be the "good" cholesterol. It is considered to be beneficial in protecting the arteries. It may actually prevent the cholesterol from adhering to arterial walls. High HDL levels are helpful in preventing heart disease.

New data has resulted in information that puts a new twist on the cholesterol debate. It may not be that the sole culprit of high cholesterol is from eating high-fat foods such as butter and eggs. There is evidence that the consumption of refined foods and the lack of fiber in the diet may be factors.

Fiber-rich foods such as oats, beans, pectins and psyllium have been found to help in lowering cholesterol levels. Studies show they significantly lower blood fat or cholesterol levels. Wheat bran and cellulose were found to be not as beneficial as oat bran and bean foods. Insoluble fiber helps to reduce the transit time of the waste matter, which in turn means less cholesterol that can be absorbed into the bloodstream (Kritchevsky, 140).

Cholesterol is controlled by the liver, the organ which aids in removing cholesterol from the blood and returning it to bile. In the bile, the cholesterol can again be absorbed back into the bloodstream. Eating a high-fiber diet can help to reduce the amount of bile returned to the liver by eliminating more cholesterol in the digestion process and lowering cholesterol levels (Story, 138).

Increasing fiber in the diet can also help prevent heart disease. Soluble fiber such as dried beans, lentils, oat bran, barley, psyllium, gums and pectins have been found to significantly reduce the risk of heart disease. Insoluble fibers are also beneficial in that they help to reduce the transit time and remove excess cholesterol from the body.

Colon Cancer

Colon or colo-rectal cancer refers to malignant tumors or lymphomas of the large intestine or rectum. A diet low in fiber and high in fat is thought to contribute to colon cancer. Heredity is thought to play a role in the predisposition to the disease. There are differences in the death rates of colon cancer in different areas of the world. The more industrialized a nation is, the higher the rate of colon cancer. The most colon cancer is recorded in Western Europe and English-speaking nations. The lowest rates are found in third-world countries in Asia, Africa and South America. Charles B. Simone, M.D., in his book *Cancer and Nutrition,* states:

> If persons emigrate from a country with a low incidence rate of colon cancer to a country with a high rate, the higher cancer rate shows up within the first generation. Before World War II, the Japanese got the bulk of their calories from rice, and the incidence of colon cancer was then very low. Among the Japanese who immigrated to Hawaii and California after the war, a significant increase of colon cancer was seen in the first generation and more particularly in the second generation. The main reason for this was the consumption of Western foods such as milk, eggs, and beef. The incidence of colon cancer is rising now in Japan, especially among young Japanese whose diets are more like Western diets.

A healthy colon is most often determined by what is consumed. Colon cancer is most likely a result of the decomposition of bacteria, excess fat and a low-fiber diet. A low-fiber diet slows down the removal process, allowing for the decomposing material to remain in the colon and be reabsorbed through the cell walls. Low-fiber diets can also cause food residue to become hard and remain in the colon for long periods of time. If this mass contains some carcinogenic material, it could make contact with the bowel. When a person eats plenty of fiber, the colon flows more uniformly and the food digestion is more rapid. It is sensible to eat a high-fiber diet which is low in fat content. The two combined can help reduce the risk of colon cancer.

A study reported and published in 1990 involved 89,000 individuals. A correlation between a high-fat, low-fiber diet and colon cancer was being studied. Not surprisingly, it was found that those individuals who consumed more red meat and animal fat were more likely to develop colon cancer (Willet, 1664-72). Though nothing is certain, common sense tells us to eat nutritional foods high in fiber and low in fat. Our diet should concentrate on whole grains, legumes, fruits and vegetables. A fiber supplement may be necessary to meet the forty grams per day for those individuals with a genetic predisposition to developing colon cancer.

Constipation

Constipation is not actually a disease, but may lead to many health-related problems. It is a condition involving a decrease in number of bowel movements or difficulty in having a bowel movement. Another part of constipation is that even if someone has frequent bowel movements, there may be an incomplete evacuation of the bowel. Waste material can build up on the colon walls and may remain there for some time. This can lead to many different bowel disorders and other diseases. Diarrhea may also be a form of constipation. Most natural health professionals agree that it is important to have at least one bowel movement per day. Any less would be considered constipation.

There are a variety of reasons for constipation—lack of activity, medication, disease—but the most likely problem is related to the diet. The typical American diet promotes constipation. Laxatives are consumed by a great many people in the United States, sometimes leading to a dependency and nutrient depletion. A simple change in eating habits will often alleviate the problem.

Adding fiber to the diet will often end constipation problems. Studies have proven this to be true. Insoluble fiber will add bulk and start intestinal movement. The amount of fiber that is recommended to individuals prone to constipation is 40 grams per day. Wheat bran is very effective, and coarse bran is the best. A combination of fruits, vegetables, whole grains and wheat bran will help keep the colon functioning properly. Adding fiber to the diet can become part of a routine. Eat a diet high in fruits, vegetables, whole grains and don't forget the bran.

Diabetes

Today, diabetes is being diagnosed more than ever before. Some health practitioners believe the the rise in diabetes is due to the refined and processed foods common in our society. Type I diabetes is a result of insufficient levels of insulin being produced by the pancreas, causing elevated blood-sugar levels. Type II involves a correlation with obesity. The pancreas produces the insulin but the receptors do not function properly to accept the sugar.

Diabetic control is often made easier if the person is put on a high-fiber diet. Eating foods rich in soluble fiber slows the absorption of food in the bloodstream. This helps stop the swing in blood-sugar levels. Eating carbohydrates and whole fiber foods together helps blood-sugar levels remain lower. Sugary cereals and refined snacks can cause dramatic blood sugar swings because most contain very little, if any, fiber to help balance and slow the absorption.

In East Pakistan a normal diet consists of wheat, wholemeal, leguminous seeds and vegetables. Processed and refined foods are not a part of the diet. One of the lowest prevalence of diabetes is found in East Pakistan. Many see this correlation as particularly significant in the importance of fiber in the diet.

Dr. James W. Anderson, M.D., a professor at the University of Kentucky College of Medicine, has done important research on high-fiber diets and diabetes. He noticed that oat bran brings down insulin requirements as well as blood-cholesterol levels. Each participant in his study was given a very high daily dose of oat bran—100 grams, or about one cup. Blood-cholesterol levels dropped about 20 percent and patients also lost weight (Hausman, 305). Such improvements make it easier for the body to deal with diabetes.

Hemorrhoids

Hemorrhoids are varicose veins located in the anal region of the body. The veins swell and often protrude, causing pain and itching. Constipation that results in straining appears to lead to the problem. The pressure from straining can cause the veins in the anal area to swell and burst, resulting in hemorrhoids.

The occurrence of hemorrhoids seems to be associated with a low-fiber diet. A lack of fiber or inadequate amounts of fiber in the diet cause the stools to become unformed, hard and dry. Cereal fibers can help to soften stools and regulate bowel movements. Eating high-fiber foods or using a vegetable-based fiber supplement also helps to soften stools so they can pass with no strain. Some individuals who have suffered from constipation for years have found relief by merely adding fiber to their diet. This simple change can produce significant results.

Hiatal Hernia

Hiatal hernia is a condition in which a portion of the stomach protrudes through an opening (the hiatus) in the diaphragm, the muscle that separates the chest from the abdomen. Small hernias are often undetected. But larger hernias often cause digestive upset, sensations of heartburn, belching, gas and bloating. How can fiber possibly help relieve the symptoms of hiatal hernia? Rita Elkins, M.H., has done much research on the effects of fiber. She explains:

> Most medical texts will cite that the underlying cause of a hiatal hernia remains somewhat of a mystery. They do know that it tends to occur in obese people and in upper middle-aged women, and that it can result from pregnancy. It is believed to be caused by an increase intra-abdominal pressure. Its connection to pressure created by straining to move hard feces is rarely discussed. As is the case with hemorrhoids, consistently forcing the muscles to bear down in order to move the stool creates an enormous amount of pressure which wreaks all kind of havoc with living tissue. Some may claim that the link between habitual constipation and hiatal hernia has not been scientifically established. Look at the facts and draw your own conclusions. *(Complete Fiber*, 131)

Hiatal hernia is thought by many in the natural health community to be caused by what we eat and how waste is eliminated from the body. Straining due to constipation can force excessive amounts of pressure on the stomach. Cultures that eat diets high in fiber have low incidence of hiatal hernia. Eating a diet rich in fiber allows for more frequent bowel movements and shorter transit time for softer stool formation.

Hypertension

Hypertension, or high blood pressure, is a major medical concern. Hypertension is a condition where too much pressure is exerted against the arterial walls. The arteries become constricted, and the heart must force blood into the system, increasing blood pressure. This puts an incredible strain on the heart. The link between colon health and hypertension is that cholesterol build-up on the arterial walls can cause a constriction of the passageway. This can obviously contribute to hypertension.

The actual link between high blood pressure and fiber has not been given much attention. Vegetarians are known to have little problem with high blood pressure, and since a vegetarian diet is high in fiber, there seems to be a correlation. Indeed, studies have confirmed the ability of fiber supplements in reducing blood pressure.

Many health care professionals are beginning to realize the importance of a low-fat and high-fiber diet in treating hypertension. Some even recommend dietary changes over medication. Research has validated the use of a fiber addition to reducing high blood pressure. Individuals who consistently eat a high-fiber diet have lower blood pressure and are less at risk for suffering from heart disease.

Obesity

Individuals who begin high-fiber, low-fat diets generally lose weight at a slow and healthy rate. People on a high-fiber, unrefined diet absorb less of the energy they take in the form of food. Fiber increases the amount of energy and fat passed in the stools. It may also prevent the complete absorption of food because the fibrous foods pass through the bowel more quickly. Researchers are finding that obesity is not so much a problem of *how much* we eat but of *what* we eat.

Adding fiber to the diet can help overweight individuals. It aids in cleaning toxins from the body, increasing bowel movements, satisfying hunger, regulating blood sugar levels, providing energy, discouraging the formation of future fat stores and improving thermogenesis. A diet that emphasizes whole grains, raw fruits and vegetables and is low in protein and fats will help to add fiber to the diet. Avoiding refined and processed foods and using fiber supplements will help to achieve adequate amounts of fiber in the diet.

The condition of the colon can be a factor in obesity. Chronic constipation should be addressed as a potential contributing component of obesity. Cultures that eat high-fiber diets are much less likely to become obese. Fiber reduces the absorption of fat by drawing water into the intestinal system which can in return cause a feeling of fullness. It also helps to increase the amount of fat that is excreted through the feces. It helps to improve digestion and alleviate blood sugar swings. Food cravings have also been found to be diminished after eating a high-fiber diet over a period of time.

Looking for the right fiber supplement can be difficult. Adequate amounts of both soluble and insoluble dietary fiber are recommended. The best combination supplements include pectins, gums and brans. Psyllium is a great bulking agent and may boost the weight-loss process.

Ulcers

Ulcers are sores that form on the mucous membranes lining the stomach. They are often characterized by pain and inflammation. They can be shallow or deep. Most ulcers are located in the upper digestive tract and are comprised of peptic, duodenal and gastric ulcers.

Stomach ulcers usually begin when the mucous lining that serves as a protection to the stomach becomes damaged due to the breakdown of stomach acid. Stress and certain foods can contribute to the problem, and eating habits are thought to play a significant role in the incidence of ulcers. Recent research has also found that certain bacteria may cause the weakening of the mucous membranes.

Research has found a connection between a low-fiber diet and the risk of developing ulcers. Bacterial involvement may also be a result of poor diet. Fiber helps to speed the movement of food, toxins, etc. through the digestive process leaving less time for bacterial invasion. Friendly bacteria (which is encouraged by a high-fiber diet) help to add protection to the digestive tract. Fiber-rich foods also help to promote the secretion of mucin which aids in protecting against ulcer formation. Barley and guar gum have been found to help protect the stomach.

Varicose Veins

Varicose veins are those vessels which become swollen due to a backflow of blood caused by a weakening of the vein wall or valve. Blood tends to pool in superficial veins, which can cause them to become swollen, sore and stretched. The legs are the most common area in which varicose veins occur. Spider veins are a mild form of varicose veins that usually do not cause discomfort.

Poor circulation, pregnancy and prolonged standing are all thought to contribute to the problems. As with hemorrhoids, varicose veins are the result of too much venous pressure from straining to pass a hard bowel movement. This straining can contribute to the formation of varicose veins in the legs and the anal area.

The connection between fiber and varicose veins is very interesting. In areas of the world where a high-fiber diet is consumed, varicose veins are rarely seen. In contrast, the Western diet is certainly a contributing factor to the formation of varicose veins. The more affluent a community, the greater the incidence of many disorders affected by diet. One study found that the incidence of varicose veins was practically non-existent in most areas of Asia and Africa. If the main cause of varicose veins were pregnancy or standing for long periods, there should be an across-the-board average occurrence throughout the world. However, this is not the case.

Fabulous Fiber

Increasing fiber consumption should be a first priority for everyone. The facts are overwhelming as to the advantages of eating a diet high in fiber. Medical professionals should recommend the use of fiber to all their patients. It is remarkable that one simple addition to the diet can promote so many health benefits. Be aware of the fiber content in foods and avoid refined foods. Becoming aware of fiber will help change shopping habits, and that will help change your level of colon health.

CHAPTER FIVE

NUTRITIONAL KEYS TO IDEAL HEALTH

I. DIETS FOR OPTIMAL COLON HEALTH

BREAKFAST

In the morning you need all the energy you can muster just to start your day. It takes more energy for the body to digest foods than to perform any other function. Therefore, it makes sense that you eat a fruit meal or drink fresh fruit juice for easy digestion and for morning energy demands. Always dilute fruit juices with half water. Fruit that is in season and tree-ripened is ideal. It contains most of the nutrients the human body needs to sustain life.

Fruits are also cleansers. They have a high water content, which helps wash many toxins and impurities out of the system. Fruits are an ideal food first thing in the morning because their live enzymes facilitate digestion and promote energy in the body. However, if combined with other foods, fruit is unable to pass through the system as designed. It causes fermentation, indigestion and gas. Cooked fruit promotes an acid condition in the body, and thus becomes an acid-forming food. Do not confuse acid foods with acid-forming foods. Some acid foods, such as fresh fruit, actually help neutralize acidity in the body because they become alkaline-forming once they are inside.

Do not clog your body with hard-to-digest proteins and carbohydrates. During the period of time when your body is without food it goes through a cleanse. The time we sleep is a time for the body to detoxify. It is also when healing takes place because body energies can be directed to things other than digestion. Toxins accumulate in the stomach during the night so the first food in the morning should be a cleansing food. Squeeze half a fresh lemon or lime in a glass of warm water and take one hour or more before breakfast.

Some people, such as those with hypoglycemia, diabetes or candidiasis, cannot handle large amounts of fructose. They should avoid fruits with high sugar content, such as grapes, dried fruit, raisins and dates. Individuals with serious candida problems should avoid all fruit until further healing takes place. Some people who have had severe reactions to fruit found that it is the spray on the fruit, rather than the fruit itself, that causes the problems. People who cannot handle large quantities of fruit should start out slowly with fruit in the morning. It is suggested to eat half a fruit, such as a banana or apple, and see how it is tolerated.

If hypoglycemia or other health problems interfere with fruit in the morning, millet dishes are a good alternative. Millet is an alkaline cereal that is easy to digest and that is rich in protein and minerals. Thermos cooking is also good. Drinking the juice that results from thermos cooking will supply enzymes necessary for digestion.

LUNCH

Vegetables and protein are recommended for lunch. If you are not vegetarian, meat can be eaten sparingly. However, meat should be a complementary food instead of a dominating food, and always eaten in combination with vegetables. In other words, vegetables should constitute the major portion of the meal. Vegetables should be eaten raw or lightly steamed. A vegetable salad with a little chicken or tuna is delicious! As you begin to eat less meat, replace it with grains and nuts.

DINNER

Vegetables and grains are suggested for dinner as they are very compatible when eaten in combination. Vegetables contain minerals and are building foods. Grains contain amino acids, minerals, and supply fiber to the diet— very important for the health of the colon and the entire digestive system.

The Phytic Acid Myth

Many dieticians and doctors have the mistaken belief that the phytic acid content of grains interferes with the metabolism of calcium in the body. They have cautioned women not to eat too many grains. USDA studies have shown, however, that volunteers eating whole wheat in normal amounts exhibit good mineral absorption. Dr. Eugene Morris says, "The whole wheat actually contributes to the body's absorption of minerals rather than subtracting from it" (*Processed*, 89).

Another study was conducted on children who were given diets with both low and high phytate levels. During the first week of the study, calcium absorption decreased. Over the next three weeks, however, calcium absorption improved as a high phytate diet continued.

II. SUPER GRAINS TO KNOW

Amaranth

Amaranth was the sacred grain of the Aztec people. It was grown on the American continents for nearly 8,000 years, but disappeared in the early 1500s during the Spanish conquest. It is now making a comeback in North America. Amaranth is an excellent food; it is a complete protein and supplies all the essential amino acids. (Note: Presoaking and cooking grains on low heat contributes to them having a beneficial effect on the body when eaten. It helps to utilize all the nutrients.)

AMARANTH STEW

1/2 c. cooked amaranth
1/2 c. cooked millet
2 medium yellow onions, chopped
2 garlic cloves, chopped
2 medium shallots, chopped
1/2 c. carrots, sliced
1 c. cabbage, chopped
1/2 c. zucchini, chopped
1/2 c. bell pepper, chopped
1 cup fresh tomatoes, chopped
1/2 c. canned green chiles, chopped
15 oz. can whole tomatoes, chopped
4 Tbsp. pure olive oil
4 Tbsp. fresh basil, or 1 tsp. dried basil
2 1/2 Tbsp. Italian seasoning

Sauté olive oil with onions, shallots, and garlic. Add all vegetables, and sauté for a few minutes. Add canned tomatoes, amaranth and millet. Simmer for about 10 minutes. Season to taste with tamari, mineral salt, or vegetable seasoning. The vegetables should be crisp. This recipe is very rich in minerals and protein.

Yellow Cornmeal

Yellow cornmeal is excellent for the colon. It is a natural laxative and high in magnesium, which makes it useful in cases of constipation. Yellow cornmeal contains magnesium, calcium, phosphorus, iron, potassium, vitamin A, and several B vitamins. Polenta is a yellow cornmeal dish eaten in northern Italy and used regularly by many Europeans—an excellent breakfast dish.

POLENTA SUPREME
    4 cups water
    1 1/2 c. yellow cornmeal
    1 1/2 tsp. mineral salt
    1/4 c. butter
    1/3 c. grated Parmesan cheese
    1 c. garden spaghetti sauce

Stir the cornmeal in one cup of cold water. Bring three cups of water to a boil, and stir the cornmeal and water in slowly, stirring constantly. Cook for about thirty minutes, stirring occasionally. You may need to add boiling water if it looks too thick. When done, add the butter, cheese and spaghetti sauce. Pour in a 9x12 baking dish. Cut in squares to serve.

Kamut

Kamut is an ancient grain, a relative of modern Durham wheat. It originated in the Fertile Crescent thousands of years ago and has a rich buttery flavor. It has 29 percent more protein than common wheat, 16 amino acids with higher value than those in common wheat, 27 percent more lipids, 23 percent more magnesium, more vitamin E, 25 percent more zinc, and is richer in eight of the nine minerals found in common wheat.

KAMUT AND VEGETABLE SALAD

1 c. uncooked kamut	4 c. water
1 c. red cabbage, chopped	1 c. broccoli, chopped
1 c. carrots, chopped	4 green onions, diced
1/4 c. fresh parsley, minced	2 cloves garlic, minced
1/2 c. plain yogurt	1/4 c. mayonnaise
juice of a whole lemon	

Cook kamut in boiling water for about 1 1/2 hours. Cool in refrigerator. Combine all other ingredients and add kamut. Add paprika, curry powder, or vegetable seasoning to taste.

Millet

Millet is an alkaline cereal. It is very versatile, and can be used in soups, cooked with rice, and added to breakfast dishes and salads. It is high in protein, calcium, magnesium and iron.

NUTTY MILLET AND BROWN RICE

1 c. millet
1 c. Basmati brown rice
1 c. grain burger mix
3/4 c. hot water.

Boil the millet and brown rice together in 4 cups water. Mix grain burger mix and water and set aside. Then prepare the following:

2 medium onions, chopped	1/2 c. ground almonds
2 medium shallots, chopped	1/2 c. ground pecans
2 cloves garlic, minced	1/4 c. whole pine nuts
3-4 Tbsp. extra-virgin olive oil	

Sauté onions and shallots in olive oil until transparent. Add nuts and burger mix to onions and cook for a few minutes until nuts and burger are browned slightly. You may need to add another tablespoon or two of olive oil to prevent burger and nuts from sticking to pan. In a baking dish crumble precooked rice and millet, then add the onion mixture and stir well. Season with mineral salt if needed and serve warm. Serves eight to ten people.

Whole Oats

Oats are an excellent grain for the colon. It has been shown to lower cholesterol and is high in protein. Oats also contain calcium, magnesium, phosphorus, iron and manganese.

MULTI-GRAIN STEW

1 large sweet potato, coarsely chopped	1 16 oz. can tomatoes, chopped, with liquid
1/2 c. whole oats	1/2 c. buckwheat
1/2 c. millet	1/2 c. spelt
8 c. water	4 Tbsp. pure olive oil
1 large onion, chopped	2 cloves garlic, minced
2 medium shallots, chopped	2 stalks celery, sliced
1 small can green chiles	1 Tbsp. paprika
1/2 c. chopped fresh parsley	1 tsp. basil
2 Tbsp. low-sodium soy sauce	1/2 tsp. ground cumin
1/4 tsp. white pepper	1/2 tsp. hot pepper sauce

In a 5-quart saucepan combine the four grains in the water and simmer while covered for 1 hour. Sauté the olive oil with onions, shallots, and garlic. Add all other ingredients to grain mix and cook until sweet potato is tender.

Quinoa

Quinoa is a grain of the Incas. It is not a true grain but is technically a fruit. It is also a complete protein. It is more versatile than rice, and may be substituted for rice in many recipes. It is a great grain for people with allergies or those who have trouble digesting wheat. It contains all the essential amino acids and is high in iron, vitamins B and E, potassium and phosphorus. One cup of quinoa contains as much calcium as a quart of milk, and is more easily assimilated in the body.

QUINOA AND LENTIL SUPPER

1 c. quinoa	2 c. water
3 Tbsp. pure olive oil	4 shallots, chopped
2 medium yellow onions	4 garlic cloves, minced
1 Tbsp. tamari	1 Tbsp. mineral salt
1/2 tsp. white pepper	1/4 cup pine nuts
3 Tbsp. sun-dried tomatoes	1/2 cup cooked lentils

Sauté garlic, shallots, and onions in olive oil for about 10 minutes. Stir in quinoa and add water and seasoning. Cover and simmer for about 10 minutes. Stir in tomatoes and lentils. Cover and let simmer for about 10 more minutes.

Spelt and Teff

Spelt and teff are two recently revived grains. Spelt was used in Europe more than 9,000 years ago. It is high in gluten and is closely related to wheat, yet can often be tolerated by those who are allergic to wheat. Its nutrients are readily available for the body to use without much digestive work. Spelt contains all of the basic essentials for a healthy body, including protein, fats, carbohydrates, vitamins, minerals and trace elements.

Teff is a grain remotely related to wheat and is a new grain to most Americans. It is essentially gluten free, and it can be tolerated by those who need gluten-free food.

SPELT MUFFINS

2 1/4 c. spelt flour
1 Tbsp. baking powder
1 1/4 cups soy or rice milk
3 Tbsp. butter, melted

1/4 c. honey
1/2 tsp. mineral salt
3 eggs, beaten

Preheat oven to 425 degrees. Place muffin cups in pan, or grease 12 muffin cups. Combine dry ingredients together. Add milk, eggs and butter and stir until moistened. Fill muffin cups 2/3 full with mixture and bake for about 20 minutes. These are delicious with an added 1/2 cup of chopped almonds, pecans, dates or currants.

POTATO AND TEFF PANCAKES

1 c. cooked teff, cooled
1 egg
mineral salt to taste
olive oil

1 c. raw potato, shredded
2 Tbsp. grated shallots
white pepper to taste

Mix together teff, potato, egg, onion and seasonings. Heat olive oil and pour batter into pan by rounded tablespoons. Mash slightly so they can become crisp. Cook on both sides. (Olive oil is good to cook with because it doesn't oxidize as fast as other oils. Just be sure not to get it too hot. It will take a little longer to cook but will be easier to digest.)

Wheat

Wheat is high in fiber and vitamin A. It is good for the colon and the heart. Wheat is a common grain, but I wanted to include a recipe that uses the whole grain, not just the flour. That way you get the nutrients fresh and unadulterated.

WHEAT PANCAKES

>   3/4 c. whole wheat (not flour)
>   1 c. soy or rice milk
>   1/4 tsp. salt
>   2 tsp. baking powder
>   2 eggs
>   1/4 c. oil or butter

Beat whole wheat and milk at high speed in blender for 4 minutes. Add salt, baking powder, eggs, and oil. Blend together and cook like pancakes.

III. ACID AND ALKALINE BALANCE

Before we can become truly healthy, it is important to understand one of the main concepts of nutrition—how acid and alkaline balance affects the body. In order to do a proper cleansing, you must know if your body is too acid or too alkaline. If you are too extreme one way or the other, going on a heavy cleanse may create side effects. Modifying the cleanse (doing it for one day at a time, for example) will usually help balance acid/alkaline levels. Acid is waste matter that is constantly developing in the body, but when the body is healthy, the acid is carried away through the colon and the urinary tract.

Acid Ash vs. Alkaline Ash Food

Before food can be used for energy it must be digested. After digestion, food is called ash and it is either acid ash or alkaline ash. For the body to sustain life, the blood needs to be alkaline. If it drifts toward the acid side, death results. Eating an acid ash diet forces the buffering organs of the body to go into a state of hyperactivity in order to keep the blood in an alkaline state. Over a period of time, such hyperactivity can cause organs like the liver, gallbladder and kidneys to wear out. This results in toxicity and illness.

One of the reasons acid ash is undesirable is that it is low in organic sodium. Sodium is one of the major buffering agents in the body. If there is not enough sodium to buffer the blood, the body will shut down some liver cells, take the sodium from those cells and buffer the system. If that isn't enough, it will take calcium from the bones and sodium from muscle tissue and use them to buffer the body. Osteoporosis and "flabby" muscles are the result of this process. The body does what it has to to get balance in its system, but is often at the expense of body organs.

One of the jobs of the kidneys, liver and gallbladder is to reabsorb sodium from the body fluids before they are excreted. On an acid ash diet these organs are forced to work overtime. Individuals who subsist on an acid diet will be more likely to develop liver, kidney and gallbladder problems.

The high-protein diet of the average American is a major cause of breakdown in the buffering system. Protein results in an acid ash and again, the body moves into a state of hyperactivity to buffer the acid. Additionally, with high protein intake, cells become engorged with protein, endangering normal cell function. Protein also takes more energy to digest than it gives in return, so it leaves a net energy loss. Meat is a stimulant that may give an energy boost at first, but will eventually end with a let-down. It also raises body temperature, which can be dangerous for overweight people in warm weather. The most excellent sources of protein are designed by nature and come naturally packaged in the correct amounts. These sources are whole grains, legumes, nuts, beans, vegetables and fruit.

What foods are converted to acid ash? The list includes red meat, poultry, fish, eggs, milk and cheese. These products are high in protein, fat, and toxic chemicals. They also contain no fiber, which puts a strain on the colon.

What foods are converted to alkaline ash? Most whole grains, legumes, vegetables, fruit and herbs. They contain nature's own balance of protein, organic minerals and vitamins, and are high in essential fiber. It is interesting to note that countries which base their diet around whole grains and vegetables have low occurrence of chronic degenerative diseases like cancer, heart diseases and osteoporosis. Countries that eat a high-protein diet centered around meat, dairy products and refined foods have a much higher incidence of these chronic degenerative diseases.

MILK AND MEAT

Besides being an acid ash, milk is very high in calories and protein—a problem discussed previously. Most people drink milk for the calcium content, but what is not common knowledge is that over 50 percent of the calcium in milk is lost during pasteurization. Beyond that, the calcium in low-fat and skim milk is not assimilated by the body because fat is needed for the proper absorption of calcium. Another problem is that the calcium in milk is an inorganic mineral which the body deposits in the joints. For some people this can eventually lead to a painful chronic degenerative disease, arthritis.

Milk is also associated with other diseases. In countries with the highest consumption of dairy products, osteoporosis, breast cancer and kidney stones are the most prevalent. An additional negative is that dairy cows are fed antibiotics and given hormones to boost milk production. These, along with other chemicals, end up in the milk that we drink. These hormones, antibiotics and chemicals are toxic to humans, which could be one reason milk is the leading allergy-causing food.

Along with milk, meat is also high in protein and fat. When meat is cooked, an inorganic acid is produced. Inorganic acid cannot be eliminated from the body because it burns tissue. It must be changed into another form before being passed through the body. This is the job of the buffering system, which must have a good supply of organic sodium, calcium, magnesium and potassium to change the acid. After years of hyperactivity, the buffering system will finally wear down and the body will become toxic.

PROBLEMS OF EXCESS ACIDITY

- Excess acidity depletes minerals from the body. A depletion of minerals lowers the ability of the body to produce enzymes, which are necessary for proper digestion and assimilation of food.
- Fatigue can result from excess acidity, which causes the cells to slow down. Most chronic conditions result in fatigue.
- White blood cell production depends upon the acid/alkaline balance. Acidic conditions lower the production of white blood cell. White blood cells are necessary for proper immune function.
- Acidity in the blood attributes to congestive heart problems, tension, insomnia and atherosclerosis. Symptoms of over acidity are allergies, fatigue, frequent sighing, diabetes, stomach ulcers, insomnia, indigestion, headaches, water

retention, constipation, difficulty swallowing, obesity, anger, stress, anorexia, toxemia and aches and pains on arising.

ALKALINE FOODS

Grains: Buckwheat, millet and sprouted grains are the lowest.

Beans: Soy beans and sprouted beans are alkaline.

Vegetables: All vegetables, including starchy ones like potatoes, squash and parsnips, are good alkali sources.

Fruit: Alkaline fruits include apples, bananas, citrus fruits, dates, grapes, cherries, peaches, pears, plums, papaya, mangoes, pineapple, raspberries, blackberries, huckleberries, elderberries, persimmon, apricots, olives, coconut, figs, raisins, melons and avocados.

Nuts: Almonds and Brazil nuts are the best.

Seeds: All sprouted seeds are alkaline.

Oils: Olive oil, soy, sesame and sunflower are alkaline.

MINERALS AND ACID BALANCE

The minerals needed to maintain a proper acid/alkaline balance include sodium, calcium, magnesium and potassium. These minerals are used up quickly when the body is too acidic and need to be replaced. These minerals neutralize body acids and help with acid/alkaline balance. A shortage of sodium can cause weakness, digestive problems, weight loss, lymphatic problems, diabetes, and bone loss. A shortage of calcium can cause weak bones and teeth, osteoporosis, sore muscles, and insomnia. Lack of magnesium can result in weak bones and teeth, nervous system disorders, brain dysfunction, weak lungs and a congested colon. Lack of potassium leads to weak muscles (including the heart), bloating, frequent infections, constipation, loss of energy, urinary problems.

HERBS RICH IN MINERALS FOR ACID BALANCE

The minerals to help balance acidity in the body are sodium, calcium, magnesium and potassium. The following lists give the mineral followed by their primary herbal sources:

Sodium: Irish moss, kelp, rose hips, gotu kola, licorice, parsley, oatstraw, comfrey, buchu, safflower, barley grass, wild yam

Calcium: valerian root, buchu, white oak bark, pau d'arco, kelp, nettle, senna, cramp bark, plantain, barberry, horsetail, Irish moss, damiana, grapevine, wood betony

Magnesium: Irish moss, kelp, licorice, oatstraw, white willow bark, dulse, elecampane, boneset, devils claw, astragalus, siberian ginseng

Potassium: parsley, horseradish, blessed thistle, barley green, hydrangea, sage, catnip, hops, lemon grass, dulse, peppermint, feverfew, skullcap

Alkaline Imbalance

Some of the main causes of alkaline imbalance are the use of antacids for digestive problems, the lack of hydrochloric acid and digestive enzymes in the stomach, and a chloride deficiency. Chronic constipation can also be a cause. Vomiting, as in cases of bulimia, poor diet and glandular imbalance, can also contribute to alkalinity.

SYMPTOMS OF ALKALINITY

- allergies
- drowsiness
- hypertension
- chronic indigestion
- skin itching
- asthma
- bursitis
- edema
- vomiting

FOODS TO BALANCE ALKALINITY

Grains: brown rice, barley, wheat, oats, rye breads

Beans: lentils, navy, aduki, kidney

Fruit: cranberries, pomegranates, strawberries, sour fruits

Meat and Dairy Products: all meat, fish, fowl, eggs, cheese, milk,cream, cream cheese

Nuts: cashews, walnuts, filberts, peanuts, pecans, macadamia

Seeds: pumpkin, sesame, sunflower, chia, flax

Sugars: brown sugar, white sugar, milk sugar, malt syrup, maple syrup, molasses

HERBS RICH IN MINERALS TO BALANCE ALKALINITY

The minerals to help balance alkalinity in the body are sulfur, phosphorus and chlorine. These minerals are found in the following herbs:

Sulfur: kelp, watercress, horseradish, cranberry, dandelion, Irish moss, garlic, eyebright, fennel nettle

Phosphorus: blue cohosh, bilberry, pumpkin seed, yerba santa, peppermint leaf, cranberry, yellow dock, horseradish, milk thistle, siberian ginseng, buchu, ginkgo, barley grass

Chlorine: alfalfa, barberry, kelp, horseradish, watercress, dandelion, goldenseal, fennel, myrrh, mistletoe, plantain, uva ursi

TESTING YOURSELF FOR ACID/ALKALINE BALANCE

An acid/alkaline test is an easy way to determine what foods you need to eat. To do the test, all you need is pH paper, which can be purchased at a drugstore or health food store. Do the test either one hour before eating or one hour after eating for an accurate reading. Apply saliva and/or urine to the paper. Wait a few seconds, and it is ready to read.

As the paper changes color it will indicate if your system is overly acidic or alkaline. It will indicate by the colors, with 7 being neutral. Acid would be indicated by less than 7 and alkaline more than 7. A balanced pH is usually between 6.8 and 7.4. If your body is too acidic you need to eat more alkaline-forming foods and eliminate acid-forming foods until your pH test shows that your acid level is closer to a normal state.

Another reason to monitor acid /alkaline balance in the body is that any degree of imbalance could decrease the oxygen-carrying capacity of the blood. Without oxygen in the blood, energy production decreases. Oxygen, nutrients and intracellular enzymes are essential for cells to supply energy.

IV. DIGESTION AND ASSIMILATION

The digestive system is our first line of defense against disease. It is the digestion and assimilation of the food we eat that determines how efficiently our entire body works. Basically, digestion is the break-down of food by the digestive system. This process involves assimilation of nutrients by the blood and lymph vessels so they can distribute nutrients to all body cells for healing and rebuilding the body.

The digestive system is responsible for feeding the cells properly and preventing illness. Digestive problems are very common and cause imbalances in the body. Toxins are allowed to accumulate, which causes cell degeneration and oxidation. The immune system is weakened so resistance to disease is decreased. The body becomes sluggish and heavier, the skin become blotchy and emotions are unstable. Many diseases are manifested because of digestive problems.

The typical American diet contributes to diseases of the digestive tract. Partly as a result of this, over 20 million

Americans suffer from digestive problems of some sort. Half of all types of cancer are found in the digestive system. The number of television commercials pitching antacid and other related products is a good indication of the number of people who suffer from digestive problems.

Sadly, new drugs advertised to prevent heartburn will eventually just cause more problems. It is usually the lack of hydrochloric acid that causes heartburn. This lack of the acid is extremely detrimental because the stomach needs hydrochloric acid to destroy germs, viruses, bacteria, parasites and worms. When we merely mask the symptoms with drugs like Pepcid, Axid, Tagmet, and Zantac, we are simply perpetuating the problem. These drugs used to be available only through prescription for ulcers, but now they can be purchased by anyone as an over-the-counter product.

The Digestive Process

The smell and taste of food help prepare the body for digestion. Digestion begins when hunger starts the saliva glands working. Saliva is important for digesting carbohydrates. Improper digestion of carbohydrates can cause autointoxication and gas in the large intestine.

The next part of digestion involves the stomach. It is in the stomach that food is broken down by hydrochloric acid— acid so powerful it can corrode metal. Besides preparing food for the small intestine, this acid works to protect the body from all types of toxins that are constantly ingested along with food and water.

The next part of the digestive process takes place in the small intestine . There food is changed into useable materials like glucose, fatty acids and amino acids. Clearly, the type of food we eat directly determines the nutrients we will receive in our bloodstream. Digestion is completed by enzymes secreted in the intestinal juices of the small intestine. Any disruption of digestive function interferes with the small intestine's main job of absorbing nutrients. If there is a thick coating of mucus on the intestinal walls, or if the intestines are irritated and move nutrients too quickly, the body will receive very little nourishment. If proteins are not properly digested, they ferment into poisons such as phenol, indol and skatol. These are then absorbed into the bloodstream and cause a breakdown in the system. If the small intestine is healthy, however, nutrients are absorbed and assimilated at a normal rate.

The final step of the digestive process occurs when waste material is carried on to the large intestine to be eliminated. Because it is the end of a long and involved process, all sorts of problems can still occur. Constipation is generally the most common.

CAUSES OF DIGESTIVE PROBLEMS

- overeating cooked food
- not enough raw food
- wrong combination of food
- tobacco
- white flour products
- too much meat
- too many dairy products
- any imbalance in the body
- lack of hydrochloric acid
- colon and liver congestion
- gallbladder problems
- constipation
- caffeine
- alcohol
- sugar and sweets
- stress
- candida overgrowth
- allergies
- ulcers
- lack of enzymes
- hiatal hernia
- heart problems

A Russian scientist named Kouchafoff found that after cooked food is eaten, the number of white blood cells increase in the intestines. The white blood cells are part of the immune system and always increase in number when there is a need to eliminate hostile invaders. This would indicate that a diet comprising primarily of cooked food can initiate the beginnings of inflammation or disease. Cooked food places an added burden on the immune system as well as contributes to digestive disturbances. It is no wonder we have so many autoimmune diseases plaguing us today.

Eating raw food, on the other hand, does not increase white cell response. In fact, eating raw vegetables before eating other cooked foods actually prevents the increase of white blood cells. This phenomenon was discovered by a well-known Swiss nutritionist, Dr. Bircher-Benner (Clark, 56). If one eats a salad with endive or watercress before a meal, it will be beneficial for digestion and will heal and repair the stomach.

Emotional stress plays a major role in stomach digestive disorders. The stomach is a very sensitive organ and nervous problems can slow down or speed up digestion. Under acute stress, the stomach has a tendency to shut off acid production. Chronic stress causes an excessive excretion of hydrochloric acid, which can cause acid indigestion. This irritation of the mucous membrane lining of the stomach may cause ulcers, hiatal hernia or other disorders of the digestive system. It is a big mistake to eat while under emotional stress.

NUTRIENTS FOR PROPER DIGESTION
• Acidophilus is important for proper bowel function. It helps to balance the normal flora of the intestinal tract.
• Calcium is an essential mineral and if the stomach is low in hydrochloric acid, it will lead to decreased absorption of calcium and other vital minerals.
• Digestive enzymes are essential in the digestion of any food. Protease breaks down protein into amino acids. Amylase breaks down starch into sugar. Lipase functions in the

digestion of fats. Cellulase assists in breaking down cellulose. All these enzymes are necessary for the digestion and assimilation of food. They help the body to absorb vitamins, minerals, amino acids and essential fatty acids, and are useful in the prevention of all diseases.

• Fiber is essential for proper digestion and elimination of food. It reduces the absorption of fat, inhibits bad estrogens from absorbing into the bloodstream, and helps maintain a healthy digestive tract.

• Hydrochloric acid (HCl) is necessary for the assimilation of vitamins and minerals; especially vitamin C and calcium. It keeps bacteria, viruses, parasites and worms under control. If bacteria is not destroyed in the stomach, it will interfere with the absorption of nutrients. One of the primary causes of an over-acid stomach is the lack of HCl. A low supply of hydrochloric acid allows food to ferment and fermentation results in other types of acids which are many times more damaging to the stomach. It can also lead to ulcers and gallbladder problems.

• Sodium is stored in the stomach wall and also in the joints. Sodium neutralizes acidity in the body. Sodium is needed when there is a deficiency of HCl. When people lack hydrochloric acid, sodium is usually lacking as well. Goat-whey powder is the natural food highest in organic sodium. It is also very rich in natural calcium, potassium and magnesium.

• Vitamin B-complex is involved one way or another in promoting a healthy digestive tract. It assists enzymes in the metabolism of proteins, fats and carbohydrates.

HERBAL SUPPLEMENTS FOR PROPER DIGESTION

• Capsicum helps in digestion when taken with meals and promotes the function of all the secreting organs. It is a natural stimulant for diarrhea and dysentery. It has the ability to rebuild tissues of the stomach and heals intestinal and stomach ulcers.

- Garlic neutralizes putrefactive toxins and kills bad bacteria. It also eliminates gas and helps in the digestion of nutrients.
- Gentian stimulates circulation and strengthens the digestive system. It is considered one of the best stomach tonics in the herbal kingdom.
- Ginger is an excellent herb for indigestion as well as for stomach cramps. It is very effective as a cleansing agent through the bowels and kidneys. It is good for circulation and promotes perspiration.
- Goldenseal contains antiseptic properties and acts as a tonic on the mucous membrane lining of the stomach. It is very effective in all digestive problems, such as gastritis, peptic ulcers and colitis.
- Licorice helps with inflammation of the intestinal tract and relieves ulcer conditions. It has a stimulating action and helps counteract stress. It also helps in the elimination of excess estrogen in the liver.
- Papaya juice and papaya tablets are very useful between meals to coat the stomach and colon. They help promote healing of ulcers and other internal bleeding conditions.
- Psyllium powder cleans the colon and prevents constipation. It is used with a lot of water to create bulk, which helps pull toxins from the intestines. It cleans the gastrointestinal tract to provide better digestion.
- A lower bowel formula can stimulate daily bowel elimination as well as clean the built-up crust on the colon walls.
  - Avoid over-the-counter synthetic antacids. Natural remedies are found in the form of herbs, digestive enzymes, acidophilus, and activated charcoal. Indigestion, heartburn and gastritis are not really diseases but are symptoms of

abnormal digestion. A well-balanced diet is the basis for good health, and with the proper combination of regular exercise, food and healthy habits, digestion will not be a problem.

V. THE IMPORTANCE OF FATS IN THE DIET

Fats are important for health! They help balance the body's chemistry and provide padding as protection for vital organs. Fats, or lipids, provide a source of energy for body processes and they help with the transportation and absorption of fat-soluble vitamins such as A, D, E, and K. They are also a source of the vital nutrients known as essential fatty acids.

Though fats are essential to health, eating a high-fat diet usually results in numerous health problems. Trans-fatty acids are toxic, sticky substances that are formed when oils are refined. They cause clumping of the blood cells and block enzymes from producing prostaglandins. As most oils on the grocery store shelves are refined, the grand majority of us are getting more than our fair share of trans-fatty acids. When oils are heated, it further changes their structure. They do not nourish body cells but instead collect in the arteries and other parts of the body. "Bad fats" (i.e., lard, margarine, shortening, vegetable oil that has been heated) cause all sorts of other problems—they prevent the essentially fatty acids from protecting the cells; they prevent natural fats from entering the cells; they create free radical damage; they reduce oxygen supply to the cells; and they destroy the myelin sheath protecting the nervous system. A high-fat diet also stimulates the over-production of hormones, especially bad estrogen that can be harmful to the breast, ovaries and uterus.

"Bad fats" are found in all processed foods. Packaged products such as potato chips, cookies, cake mixes, french fries, breads, pies, rolls, pastries, crackers, candy, and frosting mixes are just a few of the products that contain bad fats. There is no way of knowing just how long the packaged food has been on the shelf. Fresh bakery goods can be made from trans-fatty acids and rancid grains. Even whole wheat products become rancid when exposed to air. Chocolate is high in fat and is made worse because of the high amount of sugar added to make it palatable.

A good rule of thumb is that when the label on any food says it contains hydrogenated oils in any form, that food should be avoided. Natural elements such as light, oxygen and heat can cause the breakdown and rancidity of fats. The composition of extremely heated fats, especially those of vegetable origin, will turn into cancer-causing agents by creating free radical damage in the body. Stay away from fats in which the normal, health-giving properties have been altered to the point where they actually cause damage to the body's cells. Ideally, a health minded person will not eat deep-fried foods, as these are especially dangerous. However, because we are all human and it is almost impossible to eat a perfect diet in today's world, taking essential fatty acid supplements will help offset the damage done to the body by the bad fats.

Beware of Fried Foods

Many people believe that liquid oils are healthier than solid fats. Well, this is not true when it comes to frying. Because saturated fats are more stable than unsaturated fats when it comes to exposure to light, heat and air, they are more desirable than oils for frying. However, the ideal way to prepare food for frying is to follow the Chinese method of stir frying.

The Chinese put water into the pan or wok and then the oil, followed by the vegetables and meat. The trick is to constantly stir the mixture the entire time. This keeps the temperature of the oil lower and protects from oxidation because the formation of steam helps keep air from degenerating the oil.

In many commercial restaurants and fast-food establishments, oil is repeatedly reused at high temperatures. It soon becomes hard and rancid, exhibiting a strong odor and flavor. Many toxic substances can form when oils are heated to high temperatures, trans-fatty acids being the most well known. These substances are deformed fat molecules which can damage body cells. They inhibit enzymes that cause fatty acids to be changed into essential molecules. This may, in turn, interfere with prostaglandin production and cause problems with blood pressure and normal platelet action. The body cannot utilize trans-fatty acids so they just collect around fatty tissue and the body's organs. They also take up space where essential fatty acids normally would be, and perform no useful function. Obviously then, it is best to avoid frying food. If needed, use the Chinese method, or use a small amount of saturated fat, such as olive oil or butter, heated only to a moderately high temperature.

Essential Fatty Acids

Some people shy away from anything that has the word *fat* associated with it because they think it will make them gain unnecessary weight. However, there are "good fats" and if we have sufficient intake of the those fats, it can actually help decrease our desires to eat foods that contain harmful fats.

Essential fatty acids (EFAs) are necessary for the immune system. The body cannot make them so they must come from the foods or from supplements. Leo Galland, M.D., the author of a book on children's immunity, explains the value of EFAs. He says:

> My research and clinical work, and the work of many other researchers and clinicians, suggest the key to a healthy immune system is found in substances called essential fatty acids or EFAs. Our eating patterns have changed radically over the last hundred years—so much so that today we are in the midst of a famine. It's not the kind of famine that has, historically, decimated the immunity of whole nations. That kind of famine is easy to understand: it produces starvation and a critical lack of protein for the body. (16)

Essential fatty acids are vital nutritional components that our bodies need for many functions. They are found in the seeds of plants and in the oils of cold water fish. EFAs, sometimes referred to as vitamin F, cannot be made by the body. They must be supplied in the diet. Many factors, including stress, allergies, disease, and a diet high in fried foods, can increase the body's nutritional need for EFAs.

EFAs make up the outer membrane of every cell in our bodies. They strengthen and fortify tissues against the invasion of viruses, bacteria and allergy causing substances. The health of the cell membrane depends upon adequate amounts of EFAs. The benefits of essential fatty acids on human health include:

- Reducing serum cholesterol levels.
- Lowering triglyceride levels.
- Helping to clear away existing plaque from arterial walls.
- Preventing abnormal blood clotting by inhibiting the production of a substance known as thromboxane which allows platelets to clot.
- Lowering blood pressure.
- Altering the production of leukotrienes which aggravate inflammation in the body. This has shown to be beneficial

144

especially to those suffering from conditions such as arthritis, lupus, psoriasis and other related ailments.
- The ability to help with many chronic, stubborn conditions such as alcoholism, breast cancer, cardiovascular disease, premenstrual syndrome, rheumatoid arthritis, and by assisting in the proper management of weight.

Essential fatty acids are found in both plant and animal sources. The oils of cold-water fish such as salmon, bluefish, herring, tuna, and mackerel are known as Omega-3 fatty acids. The fresh-pressed oils of many seeds and nuts, including black currant, borage, flax and evening primrose, contain Omega-6 fatty acids. Processing the oils destroys the nourishing aspects of their essential fatty acids and creates what are known as trans-fatty acids.

The Benefits of Cholesterol

The much maligned body substance known as cholesterol has received a very bad rap in the press. Cholesterol, a waxy alcohol,is actually necessary for many vital bodily functions. It is found in the bile, blood, brain tissue, liver, kidneys, adrenal glands, and the myelin sheaths, or insulating material, of nerve fibers. It helps the body absorb and transport fatty acids and is necessary for the body to synthesize vitamin D. It is also a building material for hormones produced by the adrenal and reproductive glands. The body will actually manufacture its own cholesterol to ensure a continuous supply of this important fat. In *The Complete Book of Fats and Oils,* author Lewis Harrison explains:

> There are many essential vitamins, hormones, and chemical compounds that are derived from cholesterol or that require cholesterol for their manufacture. Three hormones that are

manufactured from cholesterol are steroid (or sex) hormones, aldosterone, and cortisone. (21)

Of the steroid hormones produced from cholesterol, the best known are estrogen and progesterone in women and testosterone in men. During pregnancy the placenta will manufacture cholesterol. The cholesterol is needed to produce progesterone which keeps the pregnancy from terminating. Estrogen, progesterone, and testosterone are essential to the development and maintenance of the physical attributes associated with each sex.

Cholesterol is manufactured by cells, glands, the small intestine and the liver. It is constructed from dietary by-products of proteins, sugars and fats. If the diet contains excessive fats, especially the rated types, the body will convert them into cholesterol.

Eight foods that have been shown to lower cholesterol are eggplant, garlic, fiber, apples, beans, yogurt, oat bran and psyllium. Other foods and supplements which help are salmon oil, evening primrose oil, olive oil, kelp, skullcap, goldenseal, hawthorn berries, barley, carrots, cayenne pepper, onion and lecithin.

Lecithin is very important, to keep cholesterol in a safe condition. With lecithin the body is able to create a substance that emulsifies cholesterol. In other words, it is broken up and dispersed so that it won't coagulate and adhere to the artery walls. This naturally-occurring substance is a mixture of phosphorus and lipid fats called phospholipids.

VI. Enzymes: Essential for Life

Enzymes are essential for life; without them our body's ability to heal, and ward off disease is limited. Enzymes are involved in every individual biochemical function in the human body. They are sometimes called the spark plugs of the body. Enzymes digest food; destroy toxins, viruses, and antigens that invade the liver and bloodstream; work to rid the body of parasites and worms; and help in the destruction of free radicals before they can damage the cells. Without enzymes, the body would quickly deteriorate. Maybe that is the reason we are seeing so many autoimmune diseases today—the body is lacking in enzymes.

One of the most important functions of enzymes is the conversion of vitamins, minerals, and amino acids into vital neurotransmitters, allowing our body's to function properly. Dr. Edward Howell, M.D., a physician who has spent more than forty years on food enzyme research, said, "You may have all the nutrients/vitamins and minerals for your body, but you still need the enzymes, the life element, to keep your body alive and well" (26). The only way to get enzymes is from live food or through supplements. A mostly cooked-food diet requires a larger amount of enzymes from the digestive organs. This creates exhaustion and degeneration of the organs. Supplementing with digestive enzymes will help take the stress off the pancreas and the entire system.

Overcooking food destroys its enzymes. Foods may also be lacking in enzymes due to pesticides, preservatives, pasteurization, and water containing chlorine. As a result, the typical American diet is generally lacking in enzymes. Also, as we age our body manufactures less enzymes. Supplementing with digestive enzymes and eating raw food will build up the enzyme reserve of the body.

When the body is in a positive state of mind, hydrochloric acid is secreted in the stomach and enzymes are produced in the small intestine. But when the body is stressed, angry, or tense, enzyme and hydrochloric acid activity are inhibited.

The result can be indigestion and malabsorption of nutrients. Antigens, viruses, germs, bacteria, yeast, toxins, parasites and worms can all enter the body through the digestive tract and multiply rapidly when hydrochloric acid and enzymes are lacking. We also breathe in allergens from air pollution, and most antigens, bacteria, viruses and yeast are protein, so the body needs enzymes to digest and eliminate them.

Digestion consumes a great deal of energy and needs the assistance of digestive enzymes. Supplemental digestive enzymes should contain protease, which breaks down protein into amino acids; amylase, which breaks down starch into sucrose; lipase, which functions in the digestion of fats; and cellulase, which assists in breaking down cellulose. These enzymes improve digestion and the assimilation of vitamins, minerals, amino acids and essential fatty acids. They also help the body break down old encrusted material on the entire digestive system. Supplemental enzymes should be taken after meals to improve digestion.

Additional enzymes are needed between meals so they can penetrate into tissues and break down undigested protein. This can help prevent conditions such as cancer, arthritis, autoimmune and diseases. Enzymes affect fibrin, which is associated with the cause of rheumatic disease. Enzymes will act as scavengers and destroy the protein coatings in the joints and reduce them to a form that the body can eliminate. Enzymes need to be present in sufficient levels at all times to prevent disease and maintain vitality and endurance.

Any cleanse used to detoxify the body needs to be supplemented with hydrochloric acid and enzymes. Whether it is fasting, colon cleansing, or blood cleansing, using enzymes will speed the healing process. Plant digestive enzymes are natural, and should be used instead of man-made enzymes.

VII. Amino Acids and Good Health

Amino acids are the nucleus of every living cell. In essence, they are the basis of life itself. A proper balance of amino acids can benefit the blood, the skin, the immune system and digestive system. Health expert Carson Wade observes:

> A missing amino acid is like a missing building block. The entire structure may threaten to collapse because of a single weakness. For example, you may enjoy a corn-based diet, but corn is deficient in tryptophan, and this deficiency can cause emotional disorders and insomnia. If you add grains, seeds or nuts to corn, you will provide the tryptophan necessary for brain nourishment.

In nutritional research, amino acids were long overlooked or neglected, but today they are being recognized as a great power in restoring and maintaining health. Pharmacist Robert Garrison says, "As a pharmacist, let me assure you that the amino acids are far safer therapeutic agents than most prescription drugs." Amino acid therapy has been proven useful for many ailments such as arthritis, anxiety, cancer, chronic fatigue, candida, behavioral disorders, attention deficient disorder, anxiety, autoimmune diseases, chemical sensitivity, learning disorders, eating disorders, hypoglycemia, diabetes, cardiovascular diseases, seizures, headaches and chronic pain.

All amino acids are referred to as either "essential" or "nonessential," but these titles can be misleading because all amino acids are necessary. Most of the twenty-two identifiable amino acids can be manufactured by the body and so are referred to as nonessential. But there are eight amino acids not produced by the body that must be supplied in the diet. These are the essential amino acids—isolecine, leucine, lysine, methionine, phenylalanine, threonine, tryptophan, and valine. Two other amino acids, cysteine and tyrosine, should also be classified as essential since they are derived from the essential amino acids methionine and phenylalanine. During the body's growth period the nonessential amino acids histidine and arginine should also be considered essential because they cannot be made by the body fast enough to meet the requirements of rapidly growing children.

Two of the main amino acids are methionine and tryptophan. Methionine helps remove heavy metals from the tissues. Lead is one heavy metal which causes brain damage. We are exposed to it through industrial and metropolitan pollution. It is emitted from factory smokestacks, cars, and is present in any industrialized setting. Measures have been taken in recent years to reduce the amount of lead found in various sources, but it is still a problem.A folk remedy for accumulated lead in the body is the ingestion of baked beans. Beans contain sulfur-bearing amino acids which have a chelating effect upon toxic substances, including lead.

Tryptophan is supplied to the body by eating grains. It stimulates the production of seratonin and melatonin in the brain and helps with depression and other brain and nervous system disorders. Eating a variety of grains will help to supply the amino acids needed for the body. Some healthy grains include amaranth, buckwheat, kamut, quinoa, spelt and teff. Using brown rice, millet, rye, whole oats, and wheat will enhance health and supply all the amino acids necessary for a healthy body.

Amino Acid Profile

Alanine: The main nutritional function of alanine is its essential role in the metabolism of tryptophan and pyridoxine. It also helps to strengthen cell walls. In cases of hypoglycemia it may be useful as a source of production of glucose. Alanine has been found to have a cholesterol-reducing effect when used in combination with arginine and glycine.

Arginine: Arginine is considered an essential amino acid during the growth period as it cannot be made by the body fast enough to meet the requirements of the rapid-growth pattern of young children. It is important to male sexual health because 80 percent of the male seminal fluid is made up of arginine. It detoxifies poisonous waste from the blood and supports the function of the immune system

Arginine is a chelating agent for manganese. Combined with ornithine it is involved in weight control. It works with the pituitary gland which is the master gland involved in burning fat and building muscle tissue. Arginine is also connected with increasing the size and activity of the thymus gland in cases of stress and injury. It may also help to reduce the risk of atherosclerosis. It controls body cell degeneration, is necessary for cell reproduction and muscle contraction, and assists the body in nitrogen elimination.

Asparagine/Aspartic Acid: Asparagine detoxifies ammonia, enhances function of the liver, and increases stamina and endurance in athletes. It is believed to cleanse ammonia from the system, which builds resistance to fatigue and aids in transformation of carbohydrates into cellular energy.

Carnitine: Carnitine is considered an accessory nutrient. Its primary purpose is to encourage fat metabolism in the muscles and is also necessary for the heart, body tissue and other organs. It is synthesized in the liver by lysine and methionine, together with adequate amounts of vitamins C, B6, B3 and iron. Vitamin C is essential for this conversion process. The need for carnitine increases with strenuous exercise. It improves fat metabolism in the heart and other organs. It may also help in preventing high blood fat and triglyceride levels. Men have a greater need for carnitine than women. There is a possible relation to infertility via inadequate sperm mobility. It is an essential nutrient in newborn infants.

Cystine/Cysteine: Cystine is a sulfur-containing amino acid. It is essential as an antioxidant and free radical deactivator It is considered a detoxifying agent because it bonds to toxic metals such as copper, cadmium, lead and mercury. Cystine stimulates the body's disease fighting immune system. It is a powerful aid to the body in fighting radiation, pollution and in extending the life span. Cystine protects against acetaldehyde found in air and cigarette smoke. It works with vitamins C, E, A, B1, B5, B6, selenium and zinc to protect against cellular damage and improve the health of hair and skin. It is also necessary for the utilization of vitamin B6. Cystine is responsible for supplying over 10 percent of the body's insulin, and it aids in pancreatic health. It stabilizes blood sugar and carbohydrate metabolism. Along with pantothenic acid, cystine is used in the treatment of arthritis and rheumatoid arthritis.

Glutamine/Glutamic Acid: Along with glucose, glutamine is one of the principle fuels for the brain cells. It stimulates mental alertness, improves intelligence, normalizes physical equilibrium, detoxifies ammonia from the brain, improves and soothes erratic behavior in elderly patients, improves the ability to learn, aids in memory retention and recall, helps with behavioral problems and autism in children, stops sugar and alcohol cravings, may improve IQ in mentally deficient children, enhances peptic ulcer healing, and may be used to treat schizophrenia and senility.

Glutathione: Glutathione is a tripeptide comprised of three amino acids—cystine, glutamic acids and glycine. It helps to remove poisons from the body, protect cells from destruction, clean harmful bacteria from the lungs, and protect against dust. It also builds immunity, destroys free radicals, and works as a prevention and treatment for a wide range of degenerative diseases. Along with vitamins A, C, E, selenium and zinc it may be used to treat chronic asthma, allergies, respiratory problems, and pneumonia. Glutathione also helps protect and heal the body of poisoning from lead, cadmium, aluminum, mercury. It is a form of cancer prevention, protects the liver from damage due to alcohol, and helps to reduce alcohol cravings.

Glycine/Serine: Glycine is essential in the synthesis of nonessential amino acids. Together with arginine, glycine plays an important role in the healing of trauma injuries and damaged tissue. It is utilized in liver detoxification, promotes energy and oxygen use in the cells, is necessary for biosynthesis of nucleic acids as well as bile acids, enhances gastric acid secretion, and readily converts into serine which protects fatty sheaths surrounding nerve fibers.

Histidine: Histidine is considered an essential amino acid especially during in the growth period of young children. It is fundamental for the maintenance of myelin sheaths. It is also necessary for the function of nerve cells in the body's hearing mechanism. Histidine affects the auditory nerve and a deficiency can cause deafness and hearing loss.

Histidine is important for the formation of glycogen and is a vital component of blood. It is also involved in controlling the mucus level of the digestive and respiratory systems. Histamine is released during trauma and stressful conditions causing allergies, but as the level of histidine increases, the concentration of histamine decreases. Along with niacin and vitamin B6, histidine is considered a sexual stimulant. It may be used in the treatment of rheumatoid arthritis, cardiocirculatory conditions, anemia, allergies, and stress. It has a vasodilating action, is a good chelating agent, is effective against radiation or heavy metals, and works to heal allergic conditions. Histidine has been given to cosmonauts to protect against the effects of radiation.

Isoleucine: Isoleucine is essential for growth and chronic diseases. It is necessary for hemoglobin formation and is often lacking in the mentally and physically ill. It is used to synthesize nonessential amino acids and maintain correct nitrogen levels. Isoleucine regulates the function of the thymus, spleen and pituitary glands.

Leucine: Leucine is necessary for growth and development. It stimulates brain functions, is essential for blood development, regulates digestion and metabolism, assists the functions of the glandular system, and increases muscular energy levels. Leucine also compliments the function of isoleucine.

Lysine: Lysine strengthens the circulatory system and maintains normal growth of cells. It controls acid/alkaline balance and is one of the building blocks of blood antibodies. Lysine may lessen the incidence of certain types of cancer. It may also help to control and prevent conditions such as herpes simplex 1 and ll, cold sores, fever blisters, osteoporosis, rickets, dental caries, and digestive disorders. It also helps to regulate the pineal and mammary glands and the function of the gall bladder. It is necessary for all amino acid assimilation and also assists in the storage of fats.

Lysine has been found to have therapeutic effects on viral-related diseases. It also has the essential function of ensuring adequate absorption of calcium and the formation of collagen necessary for bone, cartilage and connective tissue growth. Before lysine can be utilized in the formation of collagen it needs the assistance of vitamin C. Without vitamin C or adequate protein to supply lysine, wounds would not heal properly and be more susceptible to infection. There is certainly a fascinating interrelationship of the various nutrients.

Methionine: Methionine is important in preventing excessive accumulation of fat in the liver It also helps to control fat levels in the blood and aids in preventing the build up of cholesterol on the artery walls. Methionine increases the production of lecithin. It is also necessary for hemoglobin blood development. Methionine contains sulphur to keep hair, skin, nails and joints healthy. It works with the antioxidant selenium to protect against cancer, free radical damage, and in slowing down the aging process. It combines with choline for protection against tumor growth. It also helps keep the kidneys healthy and functioning properly.

Methionine has been used to treat rheumatic fever, toxemia during pregnancy, digestive disorders, diaper ammonia rash and blisters. Bottle-fed babies have high ammonia content in their urine which is not often found in breast fed babies. Methionine may be the antidote. It is an antifatigue agent, works to combat stress, calms the nerves, detoxifies heavy metals, and prevents atherosclerosis.

Ornithine: Ornithine works with the pituitary gland and helps to secrete large amounts of growth hormones. It aids in the burning of fat and in the building of muscle tissue and is involved with arginine in weight control. Two parts of arginine to one part ornithine on an empty stomach at bedtime is thought to work during the night to release growth hormone by the pituitary gland.

Phenylalanine: Phenylalanine is vital for the production of adrenalin. It also enhances vitamin C absorption and needs vitamin C and B6 for its metabolism. It is necessary for the growth and formation of skin and hair pigment. It aids in waste elimination of the kidneys and bladder. Phenylalanine is being investigated as a treatment for mental disorders. It is often used for disorders such as arthritis, migraine headaches, low back pain, whiplash, AIDS, PMS, Parkinson's disease. It also works to strengthen the immune system, as an appetite suppressant and diet aid, as an outstanding stimulant, for healthy blood vessels, and in treating eye problems.

Proline/Hydroxyproline: Proline is essential for collagen formation and maintenance. It readily transforms into hydroxyproline. Vitamin C aids in the effectiveness of proline. It is useful in wound healing and protects the body tissues from the effects of aging.

Taurine: Taurine stimulates the production of growth hormone. It is synthesized from methionine and cystine It is necessary for brain development and function. It is also an essential element for infants not breast-fed since it is contained in high concentrations in breast milk. Along with zinc, taurine is associated with eye function. A deficiency in taurine has been linked to epileptic seizures and it is thought to play a role in controlling seizures. It has a potent and long lasting anticonvulsive effect and is used with B6 for seizure problems. It is concentrated in the heart, skeletal muscles and central nervous system. It helps to regulate osmotic control of calcium as well as potassium in the heart muscle. It influences blood sugar levels similar to insulin. In combination with vitamins A and E it is thought to be of importance in cases of muscular dystrophy. IQ levels in Down's Syndrome patients have improved with taurine supplements taken with vitamins B, C and E.

Threonine: Threonine improves the assimilation and absorption of nutrients. It is essential in the prevention and treatment of many forms of mental illness. Threonine is required for new cell development. It works in combination with other amino acids to improve nutrient absorption, prevent fat build up in the liver when choline is deficient in diet, and is an important constituent of collagen and teeth enamel. It may help with the treatment of mental illness and personality disorders.

Tryptophan: Tryptophan is an important element for growth of the body and cell tissues and so is necessary for healthy hair and skin. It is a factor in the regulation of sleep and mood patterns, perhaps because it is involved with the chemical messages (serotonin) sent from the brain to the pituitary gland. It also assists in the production of gastric juices thus improving digestion. Among other things tryptophan helps with blood clotting and enhances the function of the immune system. Vitamin B6 is needed to catalyze tryptophan and niacin and vitamin E keep tryptophan in the bloodstream.

Tyrosine: A combination of tyrosine and tryptophan may be a better sleep aid then just tryptophan alone. Tyrosine plays a role in the function of the adrenal, thyroid and pituitary glands. It may help to create positive feelings, elevate moods, increase alertness and ambition. Tyrosine works synergistically with glutamine, tryptophan, niacin and vitamin B6 in controlling depression, anxiety, and appetite. It therapeutically alters brain function which may make it a useful agent in treating mental illness. Some patients who had previously responded to amphetamines, responded well to tyrosine therapy. Tyrosine combined with phenylalanine may also help with weight control. It has been combined with tryptophan, niacin, vitamin B6, hops, skullcap, passionflower and valerian root to aid with alcoholism. It can be used in cases of high blood pressure, the aging of cells, Parkinson's disease, muscle development, allergies, cancer, irritability, and alcoholism.

Valine: Valine sparks mental vigor, muscular coordination, nervous system function, and is necessary for glandular function and the normal growth of cells. A deficiency could lead to nervous disorders, insomnia, and poor mental health.

VIII. ACIDOPHILUS: THE FRIENDLY BACTERIA

Each body has its own ecosystem. Trillions of microorganisms live inside everyone. They all coexist within the body and are necessary for health and vitality. Bacteria have a negative connotation because most individuals associate bacteria with infections and illness. There are some intestinal bacteria, however, that are necessary for body health and the prevention of disease. These bacteria help in extracting nutrients and protecting the body from detrimental factors. Acidophilus—one of the friendly bacteria in our body's ecosystem—is necessary for digestion and assimilation, as well as protecting the health of the intestinal tract. These intestinal microflora perform many essential functions and have the ability to change according to environmental and dietary change.

In recent years different strains of drug-resistant bacteria have emerged due to an overuse and misuse of antibiotics. But usually the bacteria in our body can coexist without causing harm. Acidophilus is the primary friendly bacteria found in the intestinal tract and vagina. They help to protect the body from an invasion of candida and other germs that invade and live in the body. *Lactobacillus acidophilus* helps by adhering to the intestinal wall and preventing disease-causing bacteria from taking hold. They cover the lining of the intestines leaving no space for detrimental organisms to reside. They also help by eating food reserves and starving out the bad bacteria, forcing them to pass through without taking up residence.

Acidophilus is also responsible for producing acetic acids which lower the natural pH in the intestines. This discourages the growth of the other bacteria which flourish in a more acidic environment. *Lactobacillus acidophilus,* along with other beneficial bacteria, produces an antibiotic-like substance that works against other bacteria, viruses, protozoa and fungi (Challem, 55). They work to protect the body from invaders.

Lactobacillus acidophilus is the most prevalent form of beneficial bacteria found in the small intestine. It is estimated that a healthy colon should contain at least 85 percent lactobacillus and 15 percent coliform bacteria. Most individuals are lacking in the necessary levels of Lactobacillus which contributes to digestive disorders such as gas, bloating, constipation, malabsorption of nutrients, and heartburn.

Acidophilus bacteria also help by detoxifying some harmful substances in the gastrointestinal tract. They also aid in the digestion of proteins—required for the production of essential enzymes made in the body. *Lactobacillus acidophilus* also helps to manufacture B vitamins such as B1, B2, B3, B12 and folic acid.

The intestinal flora can be affected by various elements. The overuse of antibiotics, oral contraceptives, excessive sugar consumption, aspirin, antihistamines, cortisone, prednisone, coffee and stress can all contribute to an imbalance in the bacterial flora of the gastrointestinal tract. When the friendly bacteria are outnumbered, detrimental substances may not be excreted from the body and unhealthy conditions result. We come into contact with harmful bacteria on a daily basis. When *Lactobacillus acidophilus* is flourishing in the digestive tract, we have an added protection from infection and disease.

Antibiotics: Friend or Foe?

There is no doubt that antibiotics have saved numerous lives since their development. But many health-care providers in the past have seen them as a panacea for virtually every ailment, including viral infections that are not at all affected by antibiotic therapy. Antibiotics have been overused with disastrous results. While they are used to help the body in fighting infection, unfortunately they may also encourage recurrent infections caused by their destruction of all bacteria in the body—the good as well as the bad. This lowers the immune function and leads to a dependence on antibiotics. Because of an overuse and misuse of antibiotics some forms of bacteria are now resistant to them. Diseases which were aided with antibiotic therapy are now often resistant to the treatment.

The negative affects of antibiotics are well-known. Antibiotics interfere with the growth of bacteria, but bacteria are crafty creatures and have the ability to change their chemistry and genes to avoid destruction by antibiotics. They grow at such a rapid rate that a whole generation of drug-resistant strains can develop in a relatively short period of time. Alexander Fleming, the man who discovered penicillin, warned of the problems that could occur with resistant strains of bacteria if antibiotics were overused. He understood that the weaker bacteria would be killed while the stronger would endure. This causes strong, resistant bacteria to invade and take hold in the body.

Mitchell L. Cohen, a researcher with the National Center for Infectious Diseases at the Centers for Disease Control, issued this warning about antibiotics in 1992:

> Unless currently effective antimicrobial agents can be successfully preserved and the transmission of drug-resistant organisms curtailed, the post-antimicrobial era may be rapidly approaching in which infectious disease ward housing untreatable conditions will again be seen. Patients, doctors, scientists and public health officials must all play their part in finding ways to reduce reliance upon antibiotics. (Schmidt, 14-15)

When taking antibiotics, *Lactobacillus acidophilus* can be taken by mouth to help restore normal intestinal flora. Acidophilus will not interfere with the effectiveness of the antibiotics but protects and aids in the healing process, and helps to fight the bad bacteria and organisms that invade the body. Antibiotic use should be minimized; use them only when they are essential to health and survival. Remember that the beneficial bacteria are the first to be destroyed during antibiotic therapy.

Nature's Antibiotic

Lactobacillus acidophilus has been found to contain antibiotic properties. Dr. Khem Shahani, a professor of food science at the University of Nebraska, explains that milk fermented by *Lactobacillus acidophilus* contains an antibiotic he calls "acidophilin." It is a powerful antibiotic with similar abilities to penicillin, streptomycin and terramycin. He actually believes that it is more powerful than the antibiotics mentioned.

Detrimental bacteria invade our bodies on a daily basis. Supplementing with either live-culture yogurt or a freeze-dried capsule may be necessary to protect the body. *Lactobacillus acidophilus* can protect the digestive system from microorganisms causing infection and disease. It is a supplement that works as "nature's antibiotic."

YOGURT

Plain yogurt is basically a combination of milk and *Lactobacillus acidophilus,* the friendly bacteria that produces lactase. Lactase aids in the process of curdling the milk and giving yogurt its tart flavor. Yogurt containing live cultures of *Lactobacillus acidophilus* has been found effective in treating vaginal yeast infections, infant diarrhea, food poisoning, and in preventing flu infections.

Yogurt must contain the live, active cultures of *Lactobacillus acidophilus* to be beneficial. The intestinal flora can be disrupted by conditions such as antibiotic therapy, stress, a poor diet, excess sugar consumption, and oral contraceptives. This friendly bacteria is not destroyed by the acidic gastric juices in the stomach and protects the body by adhering to the intestinal wall. Yogurt is a great way to add the beneficial bacteria often needed in the body. Some physicians recommend plain yogurt to patients undergoing antibiotic therapy to counteract the negative effects of the antibiotic.

Many of the commercial brands of yogurt found in the neighborhood grocery store do not contain live, active cultures. Check carefully to assure the best quality available. Most health food stores have specialty brands with live cultures.

CANDIDA

Many women are plagued with a constant battle with yeast infections. It is one of the most common reasons women visit a physician. It can be a very annoying condition, often causing pain and discomfort. *Candida albicans* is commonly found on the skin, mouth, digestive tract and vagina. Candida is a fungus found in the body all the time. Normally it does not pose a threat because the numbers are kept under control by the beneficial bacteria (acidophilus). When an imbalance of bacteria occurs, candida can flourish and sometimes lead to serious conditions.

Antibiotic therapy, oral contraceptives, douching, and female hygiene sprays can all destroy the beneficial bacteria needed in the body and allow the candida to further proliferate. Antibiotics are often used to treat yeast infections when they may be the initial culprit. Broad-spectrum antibiotics can destroy the beneficial bacteria in the vagina allowing the yeast to grow. Pregnancy can also cause disturbances in the intestinal flora. Whenever a disturbance occurs, it is important to take measures to reestablish the normal balance of friendly bacteria.

A study discussed in *Nutrition For Women* found that women who daily consumed one cup of yogurt with live *Lactobacillus acidophilus* cultures had a reduction in candida infections. The acidophilus does not kill the candida but helps to encourage an environment more suitable for the beneficial bacteria to live and grow (Somer, 382-383).

Eileen Hilton, M.D., a specialist at the Long Island Jewish Medical Center in New York, followed eleven women with chronic yeast infections. They ate one cup daily of yogurt rich in live acidophilus. During the last six months of the study, the women averaged only one yeast infection (Castleman, 176).

Other studies have also confirmed the benefits of acidophilus when treating *Candida albicans*. Using this natural treatment encourages the growth of helpful bacteria.

LACTOSE INTOLERANCE

Lactose intolerance is a common condition. It occurs when the body is not able to digest the milk sugar found in dairy products. Symptoms can include stomach cramps, gas, diarrhea, indigestion and general stomach discomfort.

Acidophilus has been added to some commercial brands of milk products to aid in digestion. The addition of *Lactobacillus acidophilus* has been found to help improve lactose absorption and reduce the problems of some people with lactose intolerance. Acidophilus contains an enzyme that may be missing in individuals with lactose intolerance. This enzyme is responsible for changing the lactose to lactic acid.

CANCER

The digestive tract encompasses a very large area of the body and this leads to a high degree of exposure to harmful substances that enter the body. Evidence seems to point to the possibility of *L. acidophilus* in the prevention of cancer, mainly colon cancer. Phyllis Balch reports that a Boston scientist found acidophilus cultures can help suppress the activity in the colon that allows for the conversion of harmful substances into carcinogens. Acidophilus produces metabolites that help inhibit the growth of bacteria that can produce carcinogens.

Yogurt with active cultures has been found to help the growth of friendly bacteria and suppress the growth of cancer cells. A study in Poland found that bowel cancer patients fed one quart of yogurt a day for two months resulted in a reduction of cancer in ten of those patients.

IMMUNE ENHANCER

Intestinal bacteria are important in preventing disease. Jack Challem reports that researchers at the Institute for Medicine,

Microbiology and Hygiene at the University of Cologne, France, have been studying the benefits of bacteria in the intestinal tract. They have found that intestinal bacteria such as *L. acidophilus* produce peptides. Peptides are made from amino acids and help to increase the immunity in the body. One study used antibiotics to destroy beneficial bacteria and lower immunity. Peptides were then introduced and immunity was improved (Challem, 55).

Besides producing peptides, intestinal bacteria works to improve the healing ability of white blood cells. "Animal experiments have found that common strains of *L. acidophilus, L. casei, L. bulgaricus* and *S. thermophilus* (found in yogurt products) enhance the bacteria-eating ability of white blood cells. In a remarkable human study, George M. Halpern, M.D., of the University of California, Davis, reported that "live-culture" yogurt dramatically boosted the body's production of immune-stimulating interferon (Challem, 55).

Other Beneficial Bacteria

LACTOBACILLUS BULGARICUS

Lactobacillus bulgaricus is another of the beneficial bacteria sometimes found in the intestinal tract. Though not always found in the body, it helps to produce lactic acid and has some antibiotic activity beneficial to health. Studies have found that L. bulgaricus can help to increase immune function, aiding in healing and the prevention of infections.

LACTOBACILLUS CASEI SSP. RHAMNOSUS

Lactobacillus casei is a beneficial bacteria similar to acidophilus. Some believe that because of their close similarities, they may have been confused in the past to some degree. This good bacteria grows rapidly and aids in boosting the immune response.

LACTOBACILLUS BIFIDUS

Lactobacillus bifidus is a beneficial bacteria found in the large intestine and vagina. It is often present in the normal intestinal flora of infants and children. For this reason, some children's supplements have been formulated containing this bacteria. Breast milk contains *Lactobacillus bifidus*. The bacteria has been found to help protect infants against intestinal infections, inhibit overgrowth of candida following antibiotic therapy, and aid in breaking down lactose for those with lactose intolerance.

STREPTOCOCCUS FAECIUM

Streptococcus faecium is another beneficial component of the intestinal tract. It helps to produce large amounts of lactic acid. It reproduces rapidly, contains resistance to acidic conditions, exhibits antibiotic activity, aids in returning the normal flora to the intestinal tract after antibiotic therapy and is heat resistant up to 90° F.

Most of the microorganisms within our bodies are not harmful. Instead, they help to control and discourage the bad bacteria from taking up residence. It is important to encourage the growth of the beneficial bacteria to ensure health and vitality. *Lactobacillus acidophilus* is an important part of the intestinal flora and is essential to our very existence and health. Benefits will be felt if the good bacteria are allowed to flourish, thus making a less hospitable environment for disease-causing organisms to live.

The most beneficial effects of supplements of acidophilus are achieved when they are taken on an empty stomach. This is when the acid level is at its lowest point and helps the acidophilus to make its way to the intestines where it can do the most good.

CHAPTER SIX

Cleansing Programs for a Healthy Body

In order to make health a way of life, our eating patterns need to change. Poor eating habits are the main reason the body is laden with toxins and poisons and thus made susceptible to disease. Poor eating contributes to the key causes of disease, which are 1) autointoxication from a congested colon; 2) nutritional deficiency; 3) inherited weakness; and 4) a negative attitude. The body is amazing in its ability to overcome disease and heal itself, but a cleansing and eliminating program is necessary to retain health and allow the body to heal.

I. LISTEN TO YOUR BODY

The body has a built-in system to protect its health. It alerts us to problems and has the remarkable ability to adapt and compensate for any imbalance while healing is taking place. Any severe stress, be it physical, emotional or mental, takes a toll on health. The body needs extra rest during stressful periods in order to rebuild, repair and rejuvenate. When an individual is ill, there may be a loss of appetite, but this is part of the healing process. The body then devotes its energy to overcoming the sickness instead of using energy reserves to digest food.

When blood-sugar levels drop due to faulty eating habits, the result is often a craving for fruit. Fruit contains natural sugars which elevate the blood-sugar level slowly and safely. The body is a sensitive apparatus which will instinctively tell you what it needs. When something is out of balance, your body gives a signal, but it is up to you to read it correctly. You must learn about your body and be in tune with its signs and the signals. If you become familiar with your feelings and correctly interpret them, you can stop a problem before it becomes too serious.

Sometimes a person has to explore many possibilities before the cause of a problem is located. For instance, if you are chronically tired and depressed, you should evaluate your eating habits. You may have a deficiency of iron, B-complex vitamins, or other vitamins or minerals. If this is the case, a good natural vitamin and mineral supplement may perk you up. Another possibility is that a toxic colon is the cause, or perhaps it is allergies. Cleansing and building the body will fortify the mucous membranes to prevent allergic reactions and will also aid enzymes in eliminating the cause of allergies. The answer to any health concern lies in understanding the problem and "nipping it in the bud." Try listening to your body.

Why Detoxify and Cleanse?

Everyone needs to detoxify at one time or another. Every day we are bombarded with chemicals that are a threat to our health. More chemicals are produced today than any other time in history and many are toxic to the human body. They are found in food, water and air and have strong, adverse effects on body systems. Good examples of toxic substances are the chlorine in water and the bleached, refined white flour in many baked products. Both these substances can lead to the destruction of body organs.

Other toxins are mercury, aluminum, lead, cadmium, and other metals that interfere with neurological functions. Free radical damage from rancid oils and chemicals also destroys cells. Chemicals we ingest such as white sugar, NutraSweet®, and MSG are all harmful to the body. We also have to worry about deadly viruses. Parasites can invade the body and cause many problems. Today there are common autoimmune diseases that were never even heard of twenty-five years ago. As we understand the dangers that surround us, the necessity for cleansing and detoxifying the body becomes obvious. The following are a summary of the reasons to constantly strive for regular detoxifying cleanses:

1. To help control normal weight
2. To purify body organs
3. To treat diseases
4. To prevent diseases
5. To rest the digestive system
6. To stimulate brain function
7. To eliminate parasites and worms
8. To rejuvenate the spirit
9. To overcome emotional attachment to food
10. To protect the lungs from air pollution
11. To clean and detoxify the colon
12. To lower cholesterol
13. To lower blood pressure

II. Transition Diet

A transition diet is helpful when a person has regularly eaten meat, sugar, salt, white flour products, and very few grains, beans, vegetables, fruits, sprouts, seeds or nuts. In other words, a transition diet helps with the change from an unhealthy diet to a healthy diet. If a person has regularly eaten natural food, a cleansing program is much easier to follow.

Changing eating habits is very hard to do, and few people are willing to undergo this change until they are forced to in order to save their lives. How much easier it would be if a change took place before serious illness strikes. The food we eat and drink either acts to stimulate or to slow down the body processes. Meat, chocolate and caffeine drinks are stimulants. Sugar also creates a stimulant feeling but is often followed by low blood sugar which can lead to depression. Heavy foods can also cause the body to slow down or feel sluggish.

In order to rebalance the body the cells need to be cleansed of food residue that has collected through the years. And it takes time to clean the colon, blood, liver, and kidneys and to build up the immune system. If the body is weak, it is better to build it up with nourishing food, vitamins, minerals and appropriate herbs before attempting to cleanse. When the body is strong enough, a cleansing program can be started.

Changing our diet after years of bad habits and unhealthy eating is very difficult. We like the food we are used to eating, and many of them are "comfort foods." It is hard to change, but it can be done. Any change in diet needs to be undertaken gradually, eliminating one food at a time. Start by eliminating red meat and salt from the diet. This will begin the cleansing process. Any time a food that has been eaten regularly is given up, the body will began to cleanse. If it is red meat, for example, the body will start eliminating uric acid, ammonia, indole indican, skatole and indican—toxins from meat which accumulate in the cells. As foods are eliminated from the diet, our taste for those foods will diminish. At the same time, as a more natural food diet is eaten regularly, those nutritious foods will become very satisfying. When salt is given up, the taste buds will change and natural food will be enjoyed more. Adding more brown rice and whole grain will help the transition when eliminating red meat.

Tips for Beginning a Transition Diet

- Add digestive enzymes when cooking food. This helps with digestion, assimilation and elimination of toxins from cells.
- Add an amino acid complex which will improve digestion and assimilation. This will make you feel better as you change your diet.
- Use only brown rice and millet.
- Sprouts of all types are very nutritious.
- Mung beans are cleansing and healing.
- Fruit and vegetable juices can substituted for meals.
- Add herbal cleansers for the colon, blood and liver before meals to help the body eliminate waste material.
- Take digestive enzymes between meals.
- Amino acid drink formulas can be substituted for meals.
- Digestive enzyme and amino acid supplements between meals can help eliminate undigested protein, bacteria, viruses, worms and parasites.
- Herbs and nutritional supplements help to build and strengthen the body. Herbs will always speed the cleansing process.

SUGGESTED TRANSITION DIET MENU

Before breakfast you can use supplements that are needed for whatever condition you have. If you have candida, take acidophilus first thing in the morning (on an empty stomach) and use appropriate nutrients, foods and herbs that go along with candida. If you have hypoglycemia, eat the appropriate diet, along with supplements and herbs to strengthen the body and overcome this condition.

Breakfast first thing in the morning should consist of fruits such as cantaloupe, watermelon, peaches, grapes, pears, apricots, apples or citrus fruit. After an hour you can eat a thermos cereal, a millet or a brown rice dish or a protein drink. Fresh fruit juices or vegetable juices can also be used, and they should always be diluted with half pure water.

Lunch should consist of salads using sprouts of all kinds, grain soups, steamed and raw vegetables. Use brown rice and millet dishes. You can also drink fresh tomato-vegetable juices.

Dinner should be lighter than breakfast and lunch. You can drink fresh vegetable juices, steamed vegetables, baked potatoes, brown rice and millet dishes along with fresh salads.

III. Cleansing Diets

Cleansing Diet #1

Cleansing diets are most beneficial when used with lower bowel formulas, blood cleansers and herbs to strengthen weak parts of the body. If the heart needs strengthening, use formulas with hawthorne and other herbs for the heart. If the lungs are weak, use formulas with fenugreek, yerba santa and hyssop.

If the eyes are weak, use formulas with bilberry. If the liver is congested, use formulas with dandelion, red beet root, and milk thistle. If the kidneys are weak, use formulas with parsley, marshmallow, uva ursi, cranberry or watermelon seeds. The adrenals need licorice, the thyroid needs kelp, and the pituitary needs alfalfa. The female glands need black cohosh and dong quai. The male glands need ginseng and saw palmetto.

This first diet we present comes from the Seneca Indians. It is beneficial because during the first day the colon is cleansed. The second day toxins are released as salt and excessive calcium deposits in the muscles, tissues and organs are eliminated. During the third day the digestive tract is supplied with healthy, mineral-rich bulk. The fourth day the blood, lymph and organs are cleaned. The key is to drink only the rich mineral broth all day.

FIRST DAY: Eat fruit—all you want. Apples, berries, watermelon, pears, cherries, apricots are fine, but do not eat bananas.

SECOND DAY: Drink all the herb teas you want. Chamomile, raspberry, spearmint, hyssop, pau d'arco, and red clover blends are all excellent choices. If you sweeten the tea, use pure maple syrup.

THIRD DAY: Eat all the vegetables you want. Eat them raw, steamed or both.

FOURTH DAY: Make a pan of vegetable broth using cauliflower, cabbage, onion, green pepper, parsley, or whatever you have on hand. Season with natural salt or vegetable

Cleansing Diet #2—Juice Cleansing Diet

Fresh fruit and vegetables are rich in vitamins, minerals and live enzymes. The enzymes in the fresh juices enable the body to easily assimilate rich nutrients. Enzymes are essential for proper digestion and assimilation and they give the body the energy it needs to heal itself. Always dilute juices with half water because of the concentration of sugar in them.

Juices should be used often in our diets, but they are especially beneficial when cleansing the body. Fruit juices function mainly as cleansers while vegetable juices function mainly as builders. When juices are used during a cleansing diet they clean and strengthen the body.

Juice fasting is one of the oldest ways of healing and cleansing the body of diseases and build-up of mucus and toxins. Juice fasting helps restore the body to health as well as rejuvenate the system. This method of fasting is safer than water fasting because poisons are reduced into the system more slowly. Fruit juices are best used in the mornings while vegetable juices can be used for lunch and dinner.

SUGGESTED JUICE FAST

Before breakfast drink a scoop of fiber formula mixed with a glass of pure water, and follow with another glass of water. Also take two lower bowel formulas and two blood cleansing formulas. (Capsule form is the easiest way.)

BREAKFAST

For breakfast, eat fruit or drink juice. Included here are recipes for two different breakfast drinks.

1. 2 slices fresh pineapple
   1 bunch concord grapes
   1/2 green apple
   1 1/2 fresh lemon juice
   1 tsp. fresh grated ginger

2. 2 oranges
    1/2 apple
    1/2 fresh lime juice
    1 tsp. fresh grated ginger

LUNCH

Vegetable juices are good for lunch. Given here are two tasty possibilities. Before lunch, drink a fiber formula in a large glass of water, followed by another glass of water. Take two lower bowel formulas and two blood cleansing formulas.

1. 6 fresh carrots
    3 stalks celery
    handful parsley
    1/2 clove garlic

2. handful endives
    6 carrots
    3 stalks celery
    1/2 cup cabbage

SUPPER

Before bed, take two lower bowel formulas and two blood cleansers with a cup of herbal cleansing tea. If the cleansing doesn't seem to move the colon contents, you can always increase the lower bowel formula. Take four and if that doesn't seem to work, take six, or eight, until the colon starts to loosen and empty its contents.

1. 1 tsp. grated ginger
    1 beet
    6 carrots
    2 stalks celery

2.   handful parsley
        1 clove garlic
        6 carrots
        3 stalks celery

IV. DIETS FOR THE LIVER

The liver is the key channel of elimination. It is one of the most important organs in the body and is too often the last to be considered when it comes to health. We have to understand that good health is impossible without proper liver function, but the liver cannot function properly when poor digestion is a problem or when the colon is congested.

The typical American diet contributes to a damaged or dysfunctional liver with its high meat and high-fat content, as well as its overload of sugar and "white" products. Dr. A. Vogel, an herbalist for over sixty years, states, "Everything that enters the liver through the portal-vein must be detoxified and transformed. This is the reason proper liver function is so enormously important for the health of the whole body—more important than is generally presumed."

To underscore the importance of the liver, Dr. Vogel goes on to explain:

> There are several well-known cancer researchers who, on the basis of their experience, affirm that cancer cannot develop in the body, nor can other cell degenerations occur if the liver is functioning in an efficient, healthy way. Usually, a reduction of the liver activity is at the basis of the formation of tumors, when the purification and regeneration of this vital organ is not working satisfactorily.

Everything we breathe, eat and absorb through our skin is purified and refined in the liver. The heavy metals we breathe and the drugs we take are the most destructive elements that the liver has to deal with. Medications such as pain killers and sleeping pills are a heavy burden on the liver. The side effects from drugs have a profound effect on all the other intestinal organs, as well as the liver itself. When the liver is overburdened trying to expel poisons, the kidneys, where toxins are ultimately expelled, are also greatly taxed. If the kidneys are overburdened then the gases and toxins go to the lungs and cause respiratory problems.

Liver injury can cause vague symptoms such as digestive problems, constipation, low energy output, and allergies. Hayfever is caused by the inability of the liver to detoxify harmful substances. Liver dysfunction can also cause mental disturbances because the liver is unable to detoxify excess hormones which enter the bloodstream and travel to the brain. A healthy liver inactivates hormones when they are no longer needed. Toxic accumulation in the liver and the inability of their normal removal from the brain cells can result in numerous mental disturbances. Many ailments, such as arthritis, allergies, anemia, diabetes, hypertension, obesity, alcoholism and infertility, can be effectively eradicated as a result of liver detoxification.

A high-protein diet can overburden the digestive system and the liver. The problem with meat is that the protein does not burn cleanly. The nitrogen content in protein leaves ashes after it burns, and thus has to be eliminated from the system. With high-protein meals, the liver has to work hard to metabolize them to a simple compound, urea, which is toxic and must be removed from the kidneys. This puts a excessive workload on the entire digestive system, especially the liver and kidneys.

Many studies done on subjects who had no apparent liver damage showed that each person had degeneration of liver cells, scar tissue, a high infiltration of fat or an enlarged liver. When the liver is damaged, a lower amount of bile is produced. This causes chronic indigestion, and many people are plagued with digestive problems. Ads on television are an indication that digestive problems are widespread.

Lack of exercise has an indirect effect on the liver. It damages the liver with an overload of toxins that should be eliminated through the lungs. The excess toxins are then passed to an overburdened liver. Overeating, especially of overcooked food, puts a strain on the liver since cooked foods do not supply the enzymes and amino acids essential for proper digestion. Digestion is the most important process for a healthy liver.

According to the American Liver Foundation, liver diseases are the fourth leading cause of death up to the age of sixty-five. Yet it is not commonly known that there is a wide incidence of liver disease in America. In the past, liver damage was thought to be a problem of chronic alcoholics, but now it is seen among social drinkers, overweight individuals, people overexposed to drugs or chemicals, and those whose nutrition is not adequate to protect them. Children are not exempt, and we are seeing tens of thousands of American children with liver diseases.

Diet for a Healthy Liver

Our diet needs to be high in fresh, raw fruits and vegetables, especially greens, salads and plenty of live sprouts. Lightly steamed vegetables are also good. Foods that are high in natural sodium have been used for digestion and liver congestion. The food highest in natural sodium is goats-whey powder. The following foods are also high in sodium and other minerals: kelp, dulse, ripe olives, swiss chard, beet greens, celery, watercress, parsley, turnips, mustard greens, sesame seeds and sunflower seeds.

Fresh lemon juice in warm water taken first thing in the morning helps "kick" the liver into action. Use the juice of half a lemon or lime in one cup warm water. Add one tsp. pure olive oil, one half tsp. fenugreek powder and one half tsp. licorice root. Mix in blender, which makes it easier to drink with the oil content.

Fruit juices—especially from citrus fruit like grapefruit, lemons, limes and oranges—stimulate, cleanse and relieve congestion. Always dilute with pure fresh water; distilled water is the best. Carrot juice upon waking is a tonic to the liver and helps liquefy bile. Spinach, onions and string beans also can be eaten raw or juiced.

Steps Essential to Cleansing the Liver

1. Use a hydrochloric acid formula and plant digestive enzymes to take the burden off the liver. The hydrochloric acid formula should be taken before meals and the digestive enzymes during or right after meals. Goats-whey powder is rich in minerals, especially natural sodium, and will help heal and repair the digestive tract. Use a tablespoon three times a day.

Herbal formulas will supply nutrients to help stimulate and increase enzyme activity. The following formula you can make yourself, or find one all ready prepared. I find it easier to buy one already made up. Many reputable companies carry excellent formulas that contain herbs necessary to restore digestive health. Look for a formula that has three or four of the main herbs, two or three of supporting herbs and one or two of the transporting herbs. *Main herbs* include: gentian, licorice, goldenseal, fennel, blue-green algae, barley grass, catnip and alfalfa. *Assisting herbs* include: Oregon grape, milk thistle, dandelion, barberry, cruciferous vegetables, cardamom, and barberry. The *transporting herbs* are capsicum, ginger, turmeric, lobelia, aloe vera, papaya, and peppermint.

2. The second essential step is to use an herbal lower bowel formula. You will find the formula in Section IV of this chapter.

3. The third step is to use an herbal formula which will clean the liver, and another formula that will repair and strengthen the liver. The following will help you in finding a formula that will work for you.

Liver Cleansing Formula

Look for a formula that has four or five of the main herbs listed, three or four assisting herbs, and one or two transporting herbs. The principal herbs necessary for an effective liver cleansing formula are: burdock, milk thistle, astragalus, echinacea, pau d'arco, myrrh, chlorella or other greens, licorice, yellow dock, and schizandra. Herbs that assist in the principal herbs in a liver cleansing formula include: red beet root, parsley, gentian, horsetail, parsley, blue vervain, wild yam, goldenseal, and liverwort. Effective transporting herbs in a liver formula are: lobelia, ginger, goldenrod, prickly ash, capsicum, and fennel.

Liver Rebuilding Formula

Principal herbs in an effective liver rebuilding formula are: blue-green algae or other greens such as barley grass, bee pollen or royal jelly, pau d'arco, milk thistle, licorice, Siberian ginseng, alfalfa, and barberry. Assisting herbs are: kelp, wild yam, burdock, goldenseal, hyssop, sarsaparilla. Transporting herbs include: lobelia, capsicum, prickly ash, and ginger.

Supplements for Liver Health

- Milk thistle helps restore liver function, and should be used to prevent and heal liver damage.
- Pau d'arco tea heals and protects the liver from damage.
- Watercress and parsley tea help keep the liver in balance.
- Chlorophyll and blue-green algae are nourishing for the liver and blood.
- Germanium and co-enzyme Q-10 assist in providing oxygen to the blood and liver.
- Bentonite can be used in herbal formulas for eliminating and drawing out heavy metals and toxins from the colon.
- Lecithin is needed for healing the liver.
- A multivitamin/mineral supplement supplies nutritional deficiencies.
- Vitamin E helps in healing scars.
- Choline and inositol, found in lecithin, are strong fat emulsifiers.

V. CLEANSING THE KIDNEYS

The kidneys, located below the waist on either side of the spine, are bean-shaped organs measuring approximately 4 x 2 x 1 inches. These small organs have a very important job to perform for the body. When we have a persistent, nagging backache, we should remember that the kidneys are located close to the spinal column and the pain could be related to them. The kidneys suffer when high blood pressure is not corrected.

Each kidney contains about one million individual filtering units. These filtering units, called "nephrons," consist of receptacles (each called a "glomerulus") that are attached to tubules. Glomerulus is the name of a tuft of capillaries attached to a cupped end of a small tube. The tube that leads off from the glomerulus is called the tubule. If the tubules of both kidneys were spliced together, they would make a tubule fifty miles long. The kidney's job is to maintain a constant and healthy internal environment in the body. They adjust the body's electrolyte balance, manufacture hormones that regulate blood pressure, control calcium metabolism and are responsible for red blood cell production.

The kidneys are very smart. They eliminate whatever is bad for the body and brain, as well as an excess of anything good. If you go on a candy spree, sugar rises in the blood and often reaches a concentration too high for safety. The kidneys have the job of throwing out the excess, which they usually do quite successfully. It serves us all to not take our kidneys for granted. They are so vital to health it would be wise to remember that prevention is better than a cure when it comes to the kidneys.

Pure water is essential for healthy kidneys, but few people drink enough water. Instead, they consume large amounts of coffee, tea, soft drinks and alcohol. Even too much fruit juice is hard on the kidneys. There are also certain nutrients that are essential for healthy kidneys. They are vitamins A, C, and E. The B vitamins are also very important. Some things need to be avoided for healthy kidneys. Common table salt and baking soda are not good for the body because 99 percent of baking soda and more than 95 percent of common salt are is reabsorbed, but both are toxic to the kidneys.

Natural sodium, on the other hand, is good for the body. Dr. Bernard Jensen stresses the value of goats-whey powder as an ideal source of nutritional sodium. Whey contains vitamin B13, a carrier that guides other nutrients past the blood-brain barrier, especially in the treatment of multiple sclerosis and other neuromuscular conditions.

Kidney stones develop when mineral salts in the urine form crystals that clump together and continue to grow. Usually, under normal conditions, these crystals are eliminated from the body through the urine, but sometimes they adhere to the lining of the kidney or settle in an area where they cannot be carried out through the urine. These crystals may grow into a stone ranging from the size of a grain of sand to a golf ball.

A potassium formula is needed along with sodium to help regulate the water balance within the body. Such a formula helps to normalize the heartbeat and nourish the muscular system. It also stimulates nerve impulse for muscle contraction and helps the kidneys to eliminate poisonous body toxins. Potassium assists in the conversion of glucose to glycogen, a form of glucose which can be stored in the liver.

Herbs are also very beneficial for the urinary system. Since the kidneys are vital to life, it is not surprising that nature has provided an abundance of herbs to aid their function.

Steps Essential to Cleansing the Kidneys

1. Restore health to the kidneys with minerals. Using an herbal potassium formula and goats-whey powder will heal the entire digestive tract as well as the kidneys. Potassium formulas should contain some of the following: wild cabbage, horseradish, horsetail, dulse, kelp, watercress, parsley and barley grass.

2. Clean the kidneys with an herbal formula. Look for three or four main herbs, two or three supporting herbs and one or two transporting herbs. *Main herbs* are oatstraw, cornsilk, uva ursi, goldenseal, pau d'arco, dandelion, horsetail, juniper, cranberry powder, and watermelon seeds. *Assisting herbs*

include marshmallow, kelp, comfrey, echinacea, mullein, and slippery elm. *Transporting herbs* are lobelia, ginger, peppermint, prickly ash, and capsicum.

3. Restore health to the kidneys with the following kidney rebuilding herbs. Three or four main herbs, two or three assisting herbs and one or two transporting herbs. *Main herbs* include: kelp, dulse, parsley, comfrey, juniper berry, oatstraw, blue-green algae or barley grass. Some of the *assisting herbs* are uva ursi, marshmallow, cornsilk, burdock, borage seed, and plantain. *Transporting herbs* are lobelia, capsicum, ginger, and garlic.

Supplements for Kidney Health

- Acidophilus helps prevent infections and increases friendly bacteria.
- Chlorophyll and blue-green algae clean and heal infections and blood.
- Flaxseed oil, borage oil and salmon oil along with vitamin E help prevent scarring.
- Vitamins A and C protect against bladder infections and cancer. Vitamin C with bioflavonoids helps prevent the accumulation of toxins in the bladder.
- B-complex vitamins are needed every day to assist the liver in eliminating toxins. They are also good for the metabolism of carbohydrates, fats and proteins, and promote muscle tone in the gastrointestinal tract.
- Choline is essential. A deficiency of choline (which is found in lecithin) can cause kidney damage.
- Potassium deficiency can result in renal disorders.
- Magnesium and B6 can help prevent kidney stones.

VI. Cleanses for the Colon

Maintaining colon health will help protect the liver and kidneys, and prevent chronic diseases. The colon, or large intestine, is considered a storage place for the semisolid remains of our diet. Another of its functions is to absorb fluids, electrolytes, sodium, potassium, and chloride from the indigestible food residue it contains. The colon also takes up short-chain fatty acids which are produced by intestinal bacteria during the fermentation of fiber. These in turn can be used by the body for energy.

The colon has the essential function of sustaining intestinal microbes. There are over three pounds of them living in the colon. Mainly benign, they form 30 to 50 percent of the dry weight of the stool, creating its texture and also its odor. They have the job of breaking down any remaining proteins, fats and fiber from the chyme of the small intestine. The type of diet we eat determines whether friendly bacteria or unfriendly bacteria take over in the colon.

A diet high in protein promotes the growth of bad bacteria, as does a diet high in sugar, processed food and white flour products. Poor diet also promotes longer storage time of fecal matter in the bowel and greater potential for conditions such as cancer. Switching to a low-protein, natural food diet, promotes a positive atmosphere for friendly bacteria. This will help to prevent autointoxication. A 1982 article on the link between constipation and breast cancer made the following statement:

> We found that 70 percent of the women we tested had (foreign) chemicals in the breast fluid . . . the breast cells are in contact with the bloodstream, which will contain certain foreign substances absorbed into the circulation system from the skin, lungs, and the gastrointestinal tract.

Dr. John Christopher asserts that over 90 percent of all human ailments begin in a congested or constipated colon. Dr. Bernard Jensen agrees that all sick people have bowel trouble, are tired and worn out, and are laden with toxins. He says:

> Proper bowel function is an essential precondition for staying healthy, and if ill, to overcome sickness and disease, The "sewer system" must work properly or the body remains soaking in its own putrid waste, encouraging disease process and forever eluding health-building and vitality-producing forces. (*Iridology*, 44)

Just what is constipation? Dr. Christopher says, "Another common error which is held by most medical men as well as by the laity is that the stool should be "formed." This is a false notion which has grown out of the universal constipation habit which prevails among civilized folk." He goes on to say:

> The vegetarian Hindus of Armistar who live chiefly on ground wheat and vegetables, according to Dr. A. H. Browne, have "large, bulky, and not formed, but pultaceous" stools. A well-formed stool always means constipation. The significance is that the colon is packed full like a sausage and that the fecal matters have been so long retained that they have been compacted by absorption of water. The whole colon is filled, and the bowel movement is the result of the pressure of the incoming food residues at the other end. When the body wastes are promptly discharged as they should be, the colon never contains the residues of more than two meals and at the after-breakfast movement should be completely emptied so that the disinfecting and lubricating mucus which its walls secrete may have the opportunity to cleanse and disinfect the body's garbage receptacle and thus keep it in a sanitary condition. (*Childhood Diseases*, 138-139)

To determine if you are constipated take a few charcoal tablets with water before a meal and watch for their elimination. Tablets taken at the morning meal should be eliminated 13 to 15 hours later; those taken with the noon meal should be eliminated 17 to 20 hours after; and those taken with the supper meal should be eliminated 15 to 20 hours after. If you are regular, poisonous toxins will not be absorbed by the blood and into the system.

Enemas and Colonics

Enemas and colonics are very beneficial for serious chronic conditions and stubborn constipation. They are never the permanent solution to cleansing the colon, however, because the intestine can become dependent on them. The peristaltic muscles will not work as long as enemas and colonics are being used for eliminative purposes. They need to be used only for emergencies and serious health problems. Coffee enemas can help in serious diseases, such as cancer, to help stimulate the liver to eliminate toxins. They should be used only under the supervision of an expert in the field.

Acidophilus

Colon health depends on the maintenance of beneficial intestinal bacteria. The most important supplement to maintain friendly bacteria while cleansing the colon is acidophilus. Using acidophilus is beneficial because it:

• produces its own vitamins which are absorbed into the blood.
• synthesizes many of the B vitamins, including biotin, folic acid and B12.

- increases the absorption of calcium, phosphorus, and magnesium.
- helps normalize cholesterol levels of the blood.
- helps keep the intestinal tract free of unwanted bacteria.
- produces digestive enzymes.
- generates large amounts of lactase and may assist persons. with lactose intolerance.
- helps maintain bowel regularity.

Essential Steps in Cleansing the Colon

1. Follow the dietary suggestions for the digestive system. Proper digestion will help speed the colon cleanse as well as prevent accumulation of excess toxins. Blood cleansing goes along with the colon cleanse. Use red clover blends and others that will help neutralize acids in the blood.

2. An herbal cleansing tea is one way to get started on a colon cleanse. It works overnight to eliminate water retention, improve digestion, and enhance regularity. It can be used along with a cleansing diet. It is good to use when you are coming down with an acute disease. It should contain some of the following herbs: buckthorn, uva ursi, rose hips, chaparral, senna, althea, honeysuckle, chrysanthemum, ginger, and peppermint.

3. An herbal fiber formula is essential to help pull out toxins from the colon pockets and prevent further build-up on the colon walls. It should contain some of the following herbs: psyllium hulls, guar gum, rhubarb, fenugreek, slippery elm, hibiscus, licorice, ginger, aloe vera, black walnut, pumpkin seeds, marshmallow, buchu, dandelion, and echinacea.

4. A lower bowel cleanser is very important to help clean and loosen encrusted material from the colon walls. Such a cleanser is not considered a laxative. It helps clean, nourish and rebuild the colon wall for better digestion, absorption and elimination. A lower bowel cleanser should include four or five main herbs, three or four assisting herbs and one or two transporting herbs. *Main herbs* are cascara sagrada, butternut bark, rhubarb, and burdock. *Assisting herbs* include fenugreek, slippery elm, licorice, kelp, Irish moss, blue-green algae or other chlorophyll sources, or goldenseal. *Transporting herbs* are lobelia, capsicum, fennel, ginger and peppermint.

5. The following herbs should used to rebuild and strengthen the colon walls: bee pollen, kelp, blue-green algae, slippery elm, comfrey, marshmallow, aloe vera juice and papaya.

Natural Laxatives

LAXATIVE #1
   1 Tbsp. ground flaxseeds
   1 tsp. fenugreek powder
   1 Tbsp. goats-whey powder
   1 tsp. ginger powder

Mix ingredients in apple juice and drink first thing in the morning. It is excellent for the colon.

LAXATIVE #2
   1 heaping Tbsp. flaxseeds
   1 Tbsp. fenugreek seeds

Heat one quart of water to boiling, add seeds and simmer for 20 to 30 minutes. Let sit for another 30 minutes. Keep in refrigerator and use within 5 to 7 days. This combination helps with allergies during the pollen season because it soothes and cleans the mucous membranes to prevent irritations. It is excellent for the entire digestive tract and can be given to children in juices. Adults may want to add 1 tsp. licorice powder.

VII. CLEANSING THE LUNGS

The lungs carry out one of the most important functions of the body. With increased air pollution, toxic gases and waste are constantly being sent into the lungs. We need to learn more about how to keep our lungs healthy so that we can maintain a prime state of health.

The lungs are protected by mucous membranes, our "inner skin." The inside of the nose is equipped with a mucous membrane lining that has the special ability to secrete mucus. Nasal mucus performs the necessary function of eliminating dust and debris through the nose. It protects particles such as bacteria, viruses, fungi and all kinds of toxins and pollution from reentering the body.

Mucus has been defined both as a secretion and an excretion. A secretion has a constructive purpose while an excretion is something destructive which the body tries to rid itself of. Mucus becomes an excretion when the lungs, skin, bowels, kidneys and menses are unable to rid the body of waste matter that has accumulated. Mucus production then increases and takes over the work of other overloaded elimination channels.

If mucus becomes too thick, it dries out and sticks to the cilia and mucous membranes. This causes crust to build up and provides an environment for germs, viruses, and bacteria. This is usually how a cold or any other acute disease begins. When the mucus is too liquid and runny, it drips down around the cilia and a water nasal drip develops. It can drip into the lungs and lead to more serious conditions such as pneumonia or bronchitis. This brings on inflammation and is usually a component of allergies and hayfever. The thing that determines the composition of mucus is diet. Too much starchy food and too many milk products are well known for developing thicker and more viscous mucus.

Lungs and the Liver, Kidneys and Colon

The liver performs its cleansing work in tandem with the body's natural elimination channel, the bowels. The kidneys do their cleansing through the bladder and urethra. When the colon becomes congested, the function of the kidneys and liver is greatly impaired, which makes the lungs the next channel of elimination. Indirectly then, the liver and kidneys play an important role in healthy lungs.

Problems arise when both the colon and liver become congested and are unable to perform their normal eliminative function. Toxins build up and are thrown into the bloodstream. When blood becomes toxic and the liver and kidneys are unable to help, a substitute avenue of elimination must be found or death or severe illness will result. The lungs become the next channel of elimination to rid the body of toxins. They are required to take over the process of ridding the body of waste that should have gone through the kidneys. When the liver is congested and cannot eliminate properly, then the skin, which is the largest eliminatory organ, also takes over part of the cleansing process.

The lungs should not have to do the eliminating for the kidneys, and when they do it causes undue stress and strain of the respiratory system. The lungs are weakened and this can cause asthma, bronchitis, colds, pneumonia or tuberculosis, which is once again becoming more prevalent. Too many of us have forgotten that the lungs are the most delicate organ in the body and should be properly taken care of.

Respiratory System Care

The respiratory system is constructed with a series of specialized structures designed to efficiently exchange gases in the system—all with the purpose of sustaining life and body functions. Membranes of the alveola, the small sacs in the bronchioles of the lungs, must be able to expand as we breathe in and out, trading oxygen for carbon dioxide. Nutrients are necessary to maintain the elasticity of the lung membranes which are by nature very thin. A poor diet, incomplete digestion, free radicals, rancid fats and toxic air pollution can result in particles of matter which gradually clog the pores of alveola and cause the lungs to lose their elasticity. When this happens, emphysema or other diseases may develop.

A diet low in mucus-forming foods is considered crucial for those prone to respiratory diseases. The stomach and kidneys can handle just so many mucus-forming foods and when the kidneys are backed up, the lungs try to take over their cleansing job. This becomes very irritating to the lungs and causes respiratory diseases, especially in winter. The lungs are particularly vulnerable to colder winter air and any quick changes from warm to cool.

ASTHMA

There can be many causes of asthma. An attack of asthma occurs when the tubes that carry air in and out of the lungs constrict. This leads to shortness of breath, cough and wheezing. Anxiety and panic tend to make the attack worse. Fear is one of the most potent triggers of an asthma attack. It could even be caused by fear of an asthma attack itself.

Those with asthma should never use salt (sodium chloride) because it overstimulates the adrenal glands. It is considered a highly corrosive "drug" which cannot be utilized by the body. Organic salt, however, is found in herbs and vegetables and is useful and necessary to the body.

Sometimes asthma will respond well to nervine herbs. Air passages have been opened during acute asthma attacks by using a dropperful of lobelia extract directly under the tongue every 15 to 30 minutes. Fresh lemon juice, garlic and honey are also good to help in cases of asthma. In a blender mix 10 to 12 cloves of garlic, one cup of pure fresh lemon juice if your body is acidic, or one cup of pure apple cider vinegar if your body is alkaline, and about 2 to 3 tablespoons of pure honey. Keep the mixture in refrigerator and use as needed. It is excellent for all acute diseases.

BRONCHITIS

Bronchitis is an infection of the upper respiratory tract accompanied by a dry, violent, hacking cough and inflammation of the mucous membranes of the bronchial tubes. Bronchitis is a warning that a state of imbalance is present in the body. A short fast for two or three days will help the body create a balance. A cough may persist from two to four weeks as nature's attempt to expel the hard toxic mucus. After the lungs have eliminated and healed, there will be an improved state of health until the toxins become concentrated and accumulate again.

The herbs most useful for bronchitis are *pectorals*—agents which aid in pulmonary disease. Demulcent herbs should be used to soothe inflamed tissues and antibacterial herbs are usually needed to fight infections.

COUGHS

A cough is the body's way of clearing phlegm and accumulated mucus from the lungs. A cough could start from mucus caught in the throat, infection, congestion due to phlegm, or foreign matter in the lungs. Herbs are beneficial for coughs because they nourish and soothe irritated areas. For coughs with hoarseness and mucus use comfrey, fenugreek, licorice, flaxseed and slippery elm. For a dry cough, open a capsule of slippery elm and mix with aloe vera juice and a capsule of licorice root. Eat the mixture slowly and let it coat the throat. Lobelia extract under the tongue can also help control a cough. Let it slowly go down the throat. Other herbs for coughs are: blue vervain, bugleweed, chamomile, cherry bark, comfrey, horehound, hops, horseradish, Iceland moss, kelp, licorice, lobelia, mullein, passionflower, peppermint, red clover, saffron and skullcap.

CROUP

Croup usually results from a viral infection. It is a childhood disease that affects boys more than girls. It usually occurs during the winter months. It is a very frightening because it gives a feeling of suffocation and difficulty in breathing. It develops as a spasm of the larynx with a harsh, brassy, and gasping cough. There are different kinds of croup, each with additional characteristics. One is a form of bronchitis; another is laryngitis, which results from vocal edema and is usually mild. There is also a form of croup, called acute spasmodic laryngitis, which usually is associated with allergies and a family history of croup.

A humidifier with warm or cool moist air is very helpful. A few drops of a tincture of lobelia in comfrey and fenugreek teas is also good. Lobelia extract on the tongue will help stop the spasms and lobelia rubbed on the chest and back will help promote relaxation. Herbs for croup include comfrey, chamomile, hops, catnip, licorice, lobelia, mullein, peppermint, slippery elm, and skullcap.

EMPHYSEMA

Asthma and emphysema are closely related. (Refer to the previous section on asthma.) The real difference is that an asthmatic person suffers from lung sensitivity while a person with emphysema suffers from real physical change in the lungs. In emphysema, the walls of the alveola start to break down, altering the structure of lung tissue. One physician described emphysema stricken lungs as resembling moth-eaten wool.

A relationship exists between cadmium and emphysema. Cadmium is found in the atmosphere. The processes of refining metals in industry, burning modern products such as plastic, and making rubber tires all create cadmium. Cigarette smoking also exposes one to cadmium. Each cigarette contains a microgram of cadmium and inhaling the smoke of thousands of cigarettes over a period of many years can eventually takes its toll and result in emphysema.

Autopsies have shown high amounts of cadmium in the lung tissue of emphysema patients. Those who suffer more severely from the disease contain the largest amounts of cadmium. Studies show that the livers of people dying from emphysema and bronchitis also contain three times as much cadmium as the livers of people dying from other diseases. Nutrients and herbs listed in the section about lung protection and asthma should be utilized. Herbs that purify the blood and herbs that cleanse the colon and liver should be used.

PLEURISY

Pleurisy is an inflammation of the membrane sacs that surround the lungs. The pain in pleurisy is caused by the inflammation or irritation of the sensory nerve endings in the parietal pleura. It is essential to treat this sort of infection with herbs. Single herbs that help with this are boneset, mullein, and slippery elm. Blue-green algae also helps in infections. A poultice made with flaxseed tea placed on the chest can be very beneficial.

PNEUMONIA

Pneumonia is an acute infection of the lungs where the air is trapped in the lungs and there is trouble with gas exchange. The tiny air sacs in the lungs become inflamed with mucus and pus. Some of the causes of pneumonia are severe colds, alcoholism, malnutrition and foreign material in the respiratory passages. The primary causes are bacteria, viruses, chemical irritants, allergies. Pneumonia can also result from surgery, frequently causing death as a complication of a major operation.

The disease usually sets in with a severe and prolonged chill after which the temperature of the body rapidly rises to a high point. This rise is accompanied by the customary symptom of fever. Sharp, stabbing pain is commonly felt about the chest region and is aggravated by breathing. This is the reason people with pneumonia exhibit extremely frequent, shallow breathing.

Although germs are present in the body at all times, when the body becomes weak it is most vulnerable to the attack of these germs. Using the same methods suggested for bronchitis pneumonia can be cured. Enemas are very important to clean and rid the body of toxins and help clear up the infection.

Citrus juices and vitamins A and C are very important to help the body fight infection. Comfrey, chickweed, marshmallow, mullein and lobelia are very important herbs for pneumonia.

Steps Essential to Cleansing the Lungs

1. First, the digestive system needs to be improved. Use hydrochloric acid, digestive enzymes and herbs to improve the digestive tract for better digestion and assimilation. Eliminate mucus-forming foods and go on a juice fast for a few days. A colon cleanse should be undertaken to improve better liver and lung function.

2. A formula for cleansing the lungs should have three or four main herbs, two or three assisting herbs and one or two assisting herbs. *Main herbs* include ephedra, fenugreek, mullein, marshmallow, boneset, echinacea, chlorophyll or other green sources, and elecampane. *Assisting herbs* are myrrh, licorice, pleurisy, hops, skullcap, comfrey, plantain, and eucalyptus. *Transporting herbs* are lobelia, capsicum, ginger, and prickly ash.

3. Herbal formulas can help strengthen the lungs. After cleansing, a rebuilding of lung tissue is necessary. There should be four or five main herbs, three or four assisting herbs and one or two transporting herbs. *Main herbs* are comfrey, fenugreek, pau d'arco, marshmallow, blue-green algae, bee pollen, mullein, and yerba santa. *Assisting herbs* include hyssop, horehound, burdock, alfalfa, wild cherry, red raspberry, yellow dock, and barley greens. *Transporting herbs* are lobelia, cayenne, ginger, prickly ash, and cinnamon.

VIII. Cleansing the Skin

The skin is the largest organ of the body and the largest elimination channel. The health of our skin depends on the health of our inner organs. For example, if the glands in the walls of the stomach do not secrete sufficient hydrochloric acid, the skin can lose its surface acidity; this increases the chance of infections.

Digestion, assimilation and elimination are vital to beautiful, healthy skin. If the skin is abused with frequent washing with harsh soaps that are highly alkaline, all the protective oil is removed, as well as the acidity. A soap that is pH balanced will not dry the skin. It is better to use soaps containing natural ingredients such as lanolin, cocoa butter or glycerine. Avoid soaps with coloring, perfumes, harmful dyes and chemicals. Avoid face creams containing mineral oil because it will destroy vitamin A, which is necessary for healthy skin.

Proper cleansing is essential for a radiant, clear complexion. Dead cells, rancid oil, perspiration, toxins and bacteria need to be removed daily or black heads, pimples and whiteheads will form and clog the pores. A film of dirt and pollution accumulates daily on the surface of the skin. A combination of too much consumed fat and protein is the most common cause of fatty pimples, acne and boils.

When the body is overloaded with toxins, fat and protein, the kidneys, liver and digestive organs cannot process and eliminate them fast enough. Therefore, the body must expel them through the skin. In fact, the skin helps the kidneys so much that it has been referred to as "the third kidney." It works to cleanse acids, toxins and mineral wastes from the blood. Henry G. Bieler, M. D., a nutritional health doctor, wrote a book called *Food Is Your Best Medicine.* He says:

When the liver is congested and cannot eliminate, waste matter is thrown into the bloodstream. And when the kidneys are inflamed, toxins are also dammed up in the blood. Toxic blood must discharge its toxins or the person dies, so nature uses vicarious venues of elimination or substitutes. The lungs will take over the task of eliminating some of the wastes that should have gone through the kidneys, or the skin will take over for the liver. From the irritation caused by the elimination of poison through these "vicarious" channels. We can get bronchitis, pneumonia or tuberculosis. As is determined by the particular chemistry of the poison being eliminated. If the bile poisons in the blood come out through the skin we get the various irritations of the skin, resulting in the many skin diseases, or through the mucous membranes (inside skin) as the various catarrh eliminate or through the skin as boils, carbuncles, acne, etc.

SKIN BRUSHING

Regular bathing and washing will not remove the layers of dead skin. It takes a gentle and light abrasion on the skin when it is dry to rid the body of the dead, unwanted skin. The dead layers need to be peeled away so the skin will be able to breathe and live properly. This is what is referred to as dry-skin brushing. Acne, excessive dryness and excessive oiliness can all be greatly helped by this activity as it increases rapid cell production beneath the surface of the skin. It is considered to have the same body stimulation as twenty minutes of jogging or fast walking. Rubbing the skin with a turkish towel will make sure the lymphatic system and bloodstream are exercised. You can also use a skin brush made from natural bristles with a long but detachable handle so that you can reach your back. It is a wonderful feeling and so stimulating to brush just before your shower.

Skin brushing is an effective way to cleanse the lymphatic system through physical stimulation. It also stimulates the bloodstream, is excellent for poor circulation, and is a must during a colon-cleansing program because it helps to dislodge mucus. Start by brushing the soles of the feet and work up each leg, up the bottom and up to the middle of the back. Work towards the heart and bring all toxins toward the colon. Then start at the fingertips and brush up the arms, across the shoulders, down the chest and the top of the back, avoiding sensitive parts like the nipples. Don't forget the armpits—this is where glandular inflammation collects in the lymphs. Then brush down towards the colon. On the area below the navel, brush in movements starting on the right hand side, going up, across and down, following the shape of the colon. Women should brush their breasts since the action cleans and protects against lumps. The face should always be cleaned with a wash cloth or a natural, soft brush.

Another type of skin brushing is a brisk scrub done with stone-ground corn meal while the skin is wet, followed by a tepid or cold rinse. This thoroughly cleanses the skin while stimulating circulation. The natural oil in the corn meal prevents irritation and leaves the skin baby soft.

Steps Essential to Cleansing the Skin

1. Colon, liver, kidney and blood cleansers are needed when cleansing the skin. Skin brushing will help speed the cleansing of the skin. Use natural cleansers to prevent clogging of the pores.

2. Faulty fat metabolism is the main cause of most skin diseases. Foods rich in omega-3 and GLA fatty acids will help remedy this problem. All greens rich in chlorophyll, such as blue-green algae, are very beneficial. Goats-whey powder helps nourish the entire digestive tract and helps eliminate toxins. Faulty digestion interferes with healing of the skin.

Use hydrochloric acid and digestive enzymes to improve digestion, assimilation and elimination.

3. Herbal formulas can help cleanse the skin. This formula should consist of four or five of the following main herbs, three or four assisting herbs and one or two transporting herbs. *Main herbs* include red clover, yellow dock, sarsaparilla, burdock, yarrow, alfalfa, kelp, marshmallow, and sassafras. *Assisting herbs* are chlorophyll sources, rose hips, fenugreek, licorice, and thyme. *Transporting herbs* are ginger, cloves, fennel, lobelia, cayenne, rosemary.

4. This herbal formula is also beneficial for cleansing the skin. Use four or five of the listed main herbs, three or four assisting herbs and two or three transporting herbs. *Main herbs* are horsetail, oatstraw, kelp, dulse, barley grass or blue-green algae, royal jelly, aloe vera, alfalfa, and parsley. *Assisting herbs* include bee pollen, Siberian ginseng, suma, slippery elm, hawthorn, and burdock. *Transporting herbs* are capsicum, lobelia, rosemary, turmeric, prickly ash, ginger, and peppermint.

IX. CLEANSING THE CIRCULATORY AND LYMPHATIC SYSTEMS

Blood purification is the ultimate of all herbal therapies. When the blood is purified and toxins and acids neutralized, the body can heal itself from disease. The blood and lymph system carry a multitude of toxins that have accumulated from chemicals, drugs, toxic metals, and poor eating habits. Most of the toxins come from meat, white flour and white sugar products. Blood purification therapy is generally used along with other therapies, such as colon, kidney and liver cleanses.

Blood purification will affect the whole body. The basic principle of cleansing the bloodstream is to use alterative herbs. Agents used to cleanse the blood alter the character of the bloodstream because they possess certain properties which can be used to stimulate or strengthen the organs of nutrition and secretion. The body is then strengthened so that waste materials may be carried away and a supply of helpful pabulum is provided for the organism.

Removing impurities from the bloodstream is an important part of the work of any physician. Illnesses often arise because of the improper functioning of one or more organs, most frequently the secretory organs which fail to remove impurities from the blood. It is possible, however, that impurities may also arise from improper food or impure air. Changing eating habits plays a major part in cleansing the blood. In fact, when you eliminate the foods that have caused the problem in the first place, it is the beginning step in purifying the blood.

Blood cleansing with alterative herbs is intended to mean that certain herbs gradually alter and correct a bad condition of the blood. This should occur without necessarily producing evacuations of the bowels beyond what is normal. Alterative herbs help restore the toxic organs of the system to healthy action. They promote absorption of inflammatory deposits chiefly by stimulating the lymphatic glands. Better digestion results when the entire bloodstream is purified and better digestion means a healthier body.

The Lymph Glands

The lymph glands have the job of collecting rubbish from the cells and bloodstream. The lymph fluid has the ability to go deep into the tissues where blood cannot penetrate. It picks up toxic material in the form of acids and catarrh that have to be eliminated for the body's protection. These toxins are passed though the eliminative channels of the lymph glands. These glands or nodes collect the waste material and dump it in the bloodstream. Waste material are then transported to the colon, kidneys, lungs or skin to be eliminated.

Lymph is clear fluid which bathes all tissues of the body. The vessels that carry lymph fluid also carry lymphocytes, a type of white blood cell, and other substances essential for the body's natural defense system. Lymphocytes are vital for our overall health. They act like complex miniature computers, having the ability to recognize foreign matter or anything that does not belong in the body. They also provide a blueprint so that essential antibodies can be manufactured. If the body is supplied with proper nutrition these antibodies challenge and destroy dangerous material before it causes serious damage and health problems.

The lymphatic system helps nourish the body by transporting various nutrients to all parts of the body. The nutrients go directly to the cells from the lymphatic fluids. When the lymph glands are full of toxins, the body will be filled with acids and catarrh. This can promote fluid retention, loss of energy, constipation, congested sinuses, low back pain, aches and pains, and a general sluggish feeling. It could also lead to conditions such as allergies, arthritis, sinusitis, cancer, colitis, lupus, obesity and skin disorders.

The tonsils and appendix are two of the organs that protect the lymph system from becoming overloaded. The tonsils help in the throat area. Toxic material that is eliminated through the tonsils is usually swallowed and with the help of the lymph fluid is reabsorbed into the system and carried through the bowels. If the tonsils are removed, this protection is gone and any infection that enters the mouth goes directly into the lymphatic system, causing an overload for the lymph glands.

The lymphatic system needs a pumping action to fulfill its job and it cannot accomplish this alone. Exercise is the simple answer. Exercises that involve an up and down movement, like most aerobic programs or jumping on a mini-trampoline, causes the lymph vessels to expand and compress, to stretch and relax. This is an action that the lymph fluids need to do their vital job. These types of exercise will provide the pumping necessary to stimulate the fluids and help in the elimination of wastes and toxins. In *Foundations of Health: The Liver and Digestive Herbal,* it reads:

> For a lymphatic massage, oil your body well with a high quality massage oil, and then "milk" or stroke the lymphatic channels, starting around your feet and ankles, then moving up to calves, groin and into the intestinal area. Then follow a similar procedure to move lymph down from the jaw, and through the neck, clavicle, breast area, and finally into the intestines. Of course it is not only more fun to receive a lymphatic massage from a friend or a professional therapist, it will probably be more thorough.

Follow the cleanse for the blood, which will also clean the lymphatics. Use glandular herbs and blood, colon and liver cleansers. Use hydrochloric acid to ensure minerals are being assimilated because minerals need an acid condition in the stomach for proper assimilation. Use digestive enzymes.

There are numerous lymphatic vessels in the colon. Any excess water in the colon is absorbed by the lymphatic vessels. If water is lacking in the colon area, the job of the lymphatic vessels cannot continue to eliminate the toxins. At the same time it will cause constipation. Use minerals, green drinks, and a lot of raw fruits and vegetables to make sure everything is in balance.

Steps Essential to Cleansing the Blood

1. A change in diet is necessary. Add healthy foods, hydrochloric acid and digestive enzymes to improve and repair the digestive system. Improving the digestive system is the first step to help the body heal itself.

2. Occasional fasting is necessary to help the body heal itself. It gives the digestive tract a rest and with the proper herbs, healing will occur.

3. Use an herbal formula to help cleanse the blood. An effective blood cleanser should have four or five of these main herbs, with three or four assisting herbs and one or two transporting herbs. *Main herbs* are red clover, pau d'arco, chaparral, echinacea, burdock, Oregon grape, goldenseal, ho shou wu, milk thistle, and suma. *Assisting herbs* are sheep sorrel, peach bark, licorice, astragalus, hyssop, myrrh gum, sarsaparilla, dandelion, wild yam, yellow dock, and cat's claw. *Transporting herbs* include prickly ash, ginger, lobelia, capsicum, kelp, fennel, cinnamon, and peppermint.

Natural Interferon

Interferon is a natural substance that is produced by the body to counteract viruses and cancer. It travels through the blood casting its protective net over different parts of the body. It also helps to regulate other immune cells by increasing the production of fighting T-cells.

Japanese researchers discovered that a component in licorice stimulates the immune system to produce interferon. The following nutrients will help the body stimulate natural interferon: chlorophyll, astragalus, vitamin C with bioflavonoids, sea vegetables, dulse, blue-green algae, ginkgo, milk thistle, pau d'arco, schizandra, Siberian ginseng, suma, wheat grass juice, dong quai, echinacea, red raspberry, ho-shou-wu, and germanium.

X. CLEANSING THE BODY OF PARASITES AND WORMS

Parasites and worms are becoming a real problem in the United States. Sanitation measures have been breaking down and people commonly ingest contaminated food and water, or dirt. If hydrochloric acid is functioning properly in the stomach, the body will destroy parasites and worms, along with their larva. To do this, however, the body has to be free from toxins. A diet rich in fat, starch and sugar provides food for parasites and worms to live on. But a clean, well-nourished body is not an environment that will support parasites.

Parasites and worms are scavengers and organisms that live within, upon or at the expense of another organism, known as the host, without contributing to the survival of the host. Parasites take on the vibrations of the host they invade so they are difficult to detect. The danger of having them in the body is that their waste is extremely poisonous and can be toxic to the host. Some parasites act as foreign-body irritants in the tissues of the host and cause a chronic inflammatory reaction. Some worms rob their hosts of serious amounts of blood and large tapeworms deprive them of digested food.

It has been discovered that some cancers may also be caused by a parasite. Dr. Virginia Livingston-Wheeler, M. D., in her book *The Conquest of Cancer,* names the cancer-causing parasite "the progenitor cryptocide." This parasite begins as the lepra or tubercular bacillus and changes form to become the cancer parasite. She says, "This microbe is present in all our cells, and it is only our immune systems that keep it suppressed. When our immune system is weakened, either by poor diet, infected food or old age, this microbe gains a foothold and starts cancer cells growing into tumors" (5-6).

Steps Essential for Eradicating Parasites and Worms

1. Hydrochloric acid and digestive enzymes are very important. Blood, colon and liver cleansers are necessary to get rid of the toxins that parasites and worms feed on.

2. Eliminate white flour and sugar products. Eat a diet using fresh and steamed vegetables. Salads are important but need to be rinsed in apple cider vinegar to kill any larva.

3. An herbal formula to destroy and expel worms from the body should contain four or five main herbs, three or four assisting herbs and one or two transporting herbs. *Main herbs* are black walnut hulls, wormwood, garlic, cloves, chaparral, gentian, pumpkin seeds, tea tree oil, cascara sagrada, aloe vera, and licorice. *Assisting herbs* are rhubarb, barberry, gentian, blue-green algae, thyme, calendula, and alfalfa. *Transporting herbs* include lobelia, ginger, prickly ash, peppermint, and capsicum.

BIBLIOGRAPHY

Balch, James F., M.D. and Phyllis A. Balch, *Prescription For Nutritional Healing* (Garden City Park, NY: Avery Publishing Group, 1997).

Bassler, Anthony, M.D., Article published in *U.S. Medical Record* (Jan. 1, 1941).

Bassler, Anthony, M.D., "Chronical Intestinal Toxemia," *U.S. Medical Record* (Jan 17, 1937).

Bateson-Koch, Carolee, *Allergies: Disease in Disguise* (Burnaby, B.C. Canada: Alive Books, 1994).

Bieler, Henry G., M.D., *Food Is Your Best Medicine* (New York, NY: Random House, 1965).

Brown, Donald J. *Herbal Prescription For Better Health* (Rocklin, CA: Prima Publishing, 1996).

Castleman, Michael, *Nature's Cures.* (Emmaus, Pennsylvania: Rodale Press, Inc., 1996).

Challem, Jack "Good Bacteria that Fight the Bad," *Let's Live.* October 1995.

Chichoke, Anthony J., *Enzymes and Enzyme Therapy* (New Cannan, Connecticut: Keats Publishing, 1994).

Christopher, John R., *Childhood Diseases* (Springville, UT: Christopher Publications, 1978).

Christopher, John R., *Regenerative Diet* (Springville, UT: Christopher Publications, 1982).

Clark, Linda, *The New Way To Eat* (Millbrae, CA: Celestial Arts, 1980).

Elkins, Rita, *The Complete Fiber Fact Book* (Pleasant Grove, UT: Woodland Publishing, Inc., 1996).

Elkins, Rita, *The Complete Home Health Advisor* (Pleasant Grove, UT: Woodland Publishing, Inc., 1994).

Fitch, William E., M.D., "Putrefactive Intestinal Toxemia," *Medical Journal and Record* (132) (August 20, 1930).

Galland, Leo, M.D., *Superimmunity for Kids* (NY: Copestone Press, Inc., 1988).

Gittleman, Ann Louise, *Guess What Came To Dinner* (Garden City Park, NY: Avery Publishing, Inc., 1993).

Harrison, Lewis, *The Complete Book of Fats and Oils* (Garden City Park, NY: Avery Publishing, 1990).

Hausman, Patricia and Judith Benn Hurley, *The Healing Foods* (Emmaus, Pennsylvania: Rodale Press, 1989).

Hawley, Clark W., M.D., "Autointoxication and Eye Diseases," *Opthamology Magazine* 10 (14) (1914).

Hobbs, Christopher, *Foundations of Health* (Capitola, CA: Botanica Press, 1992).

Howell, Edward, M.D., *Enzyme Nutrition* (Garden City Park, NY: Avery Publishing Group, 1985).

Jensen, Bernard, D.C., N.D., *Iridology: The Science and Practice in the Healing Arts* Vol. II (Escondido, CA: Bernard Jensen Enterprises, 1982).

Jensen, Bernard, D.C., N.D., *Tissue Cleansing Through Bowel Management* (Escondido, CA: Bernard Jensen Enterprises, 1993).

Keji, C. and S. Jun, "Progress of research of ischemic stroke treated with Chinese medicine," *Journal of Traditional Chinese Medicine.* (12) (1992).

Kellogg, John Harvey, M.D., *Colon Hygiene* (Battle Creek, MI: Good Health Publishing Co., 1916).

Kritchevsky, David, Charles Bonfield and James W. Anderson, Eds., *Dietary Fiber.* (New York: Plenum Press, 1988).

Lane, Sir, W. Arbuthnot, M.D., *The Prevention of the Diseases Peculiar to Civilization* (NY: Foundation for Alternative Cancer Therapies, revised 1981).

Lindlahr, Henry, M.D., *Philosophy of Natural Therapeutics* (Chicago, IL: Lindlahr Publishing Co., 1918).

Lindlahr, Henry, M.D., *Practice of Natural Therapeutics* (Chicago, IL: Lindlahr Publishing Co., 1919).

Livingston-Wheeler, Virginia, M.D., *The Conquest of Cancer* (NY: Franklin Watts, 1984).

Michnovicz, Jon J., *How To Reduce Your Risk of Breast Cancer* (NY: Warner Books, 1994)

Monte, Tom, World Medicine, *The East West Guide To Healing Your Body* (NY: Putnam Publishing Group, 1993).

Murray, Michael T. *Healing With Whole Foods* (Rocklin, CA: Prima Publishing, 1993).

Page, Linda Rector, *How to be Your Own Herbal Pharmacist* (1991).

Pitchford, Paul, *Healing With Whole Foods* (Berkeley, CA: North Atlantic Books, 1993).

"Processed Prepared Food," *USDA Report* (May 1980).

Radifer, Leo M., PhD., "The Colon: Pandora's Box of Mankind's Ills," *The Nutritional Consultant* (Feb. 1984).

Rogers, Sherry A., M.D., "Healing From the Inside Out: The Leaky Gut Syndrome." *Let's Live* (April 1995).

Rogers, Sherry A., M.D., *Wellness Against All Odds* (Syracuse, NY: Prestige Publishing, 1994).

Rona, Zoltan P., M.D., *Return To The Joy Of Health* (Burnaby, B.C. Canada: Alive Books, 1995).

Satterlee, Reese M.D. and Watson W. Eldridge, M.D. "Symptomatology of the Nervous System In Chronic Intestinal Toxemia," *Journal of the American Medical Association* 69 (17) (1917).

Scheer, James F., "Acidophilus, Nautre's Antibiotic," *Better Nutrition For Today's Living* (August, 1993).

Schmidt, Michael A., Lendon H. Smith, and Keith W. Sehnert. *Beyond Antibiotics* (Berkeley, CA: North Atlantic Books, 1994).

Simone, Charles B., M.D., *Cancer and Nutrition* (Garden City Park, N.Y.: Avery Publishing, 1992).

Somer, Elizabeth, *Nutrition For Women, The Complete Guide.* (New York: Henry Holt and Company, 1993).

Story, J.A., "Dietary fiber and lipid metabolism," *Medical Aspects of Dietary Fiber,* (New York: Plenum Medical, 1980).

Stucky, J.M., M.D., "Intestinal Intoxication," *Journal of the American Medical Association* (Oct. 9, 1909).

Synnott, Martin J., M.D., *Intestinal Toxemia: Its Diagnosis and Treatment* (NY: A.R. Elliot Publishing Co., 1932).

Synnott, Martin J., M.D., Article in *Medical Journal and Record: A National Review of Medicine and Surgery* (Dec. 7, 1932).

Tenney, Louise, *Encycopedia of Natural Remedies* (Pleasant Grove, UT: Woodland Publishing, Inc., 1995).

Tenney, Louise, *Today's Herbal Health For Women* (Pleasant Grove, UT: Woodland Publishing, Inc., 1996).

Tenney, Louise, *Today's Herbal Health* (Pleasant Grove, UT: Woodland Publishing, Inc., 1997).

Tenney, Louise, *Nutritional Guide* (Pleasant Grove, UT: Woodland Publishing, Inc., 1994).

Vogel, H.C.A., M.D., "Improved liver function," *Bestways* (September 1986).

Vogel, H.C.A., M. D., *The Nature Doctor* (New Canaan, CT: Keats Publishing, 1991).

Wade, Carlson, *Amino Acids Book* (New Canaan, CT: Keats Publishg, 1985).

Willet, et al, "Relation of meat, fat and fiber intake to the risk of colon cancer in a prospective study among women." *New England Journal of Medicine* (323):1664-72.

Yiamouyiannis, John, M.D. *Fluoride and the Aging Factor* (Delaware, Ohio: Health Action Press, 1993).

INDEX